GOD'S PLAN FOR FIRST TIME DADS

EVERYTHING FROM
UNDERSTANDING PREGNANCY
TO NEW DAD DEVOTIONALS AND PRAYERS

BRIAN KELLER

CONTENTS

PREFACE

As you hold this book in your hands, you are at the threshold of one of life's most remarkable and sacred adventures – fatherhood. This journey you are about to embark upon is not solely a journey of the body or of the mind, but profoundly of the spirit. In the pages that follow, you will find a guide that intertwines the physical milestones of your baby's development with the spiritual milestones of your growth as a Christian.

In the Christian faith, fatherhood is more than a biological or societal role; it is a divine calling. It is a vocation that carries with it the weight of responsibility and the lightness of immense joy. As you prepare to welcome a new life into this world, you are not just nurturing a child, but you are nurturing a soul. In this book, you will learn not only about the developmental stages of your baby but also about the spiritual significance of these stages in the light of Christian teachings. You will discover how to be a mirror of God's love, patience, and wisdom for your child.

This journey through pregnancy is as much yours as it is your partner's and your unborn child's. Your faith will serve as your compass, providing strength in moments of uncertainty and joy in times of celebration. This book will guide you in using your faith to support your partner, to connect with your unborn child, and to prepare yourself spiritually for the role of a lifetime.

As we walk through each month of pregnancy, we will delve into the wondrous physical developments of your baby, while also reflecting on these milestones through a spiritual lens. You will find prayers, scriptural insights, and spiritual reflections that are tailored to each stage of your journey, and designed to deepen your experience as a father-to-be.

This book is more than a pregnancy handbook; it is a spiritual companion. It is designed to be a source of comfort, a font of wisdom, and a guide to prayer. It will support you in understanding the complexities of pregnancy and early parenthood, while also offering you tools to build a foundation of faith for your growing family.

As you journey through these chapters, you are invited to embrace this calling of fatherhood with your whole heart and soul. The path of fatherhood is a beautiful intermingling of challenges and rewards, and your faith will be the beacon that guides you through. This journey is an opportunity to deepen your own faith, to strengthen your relationship with God, and to prepare to raise your child in a home filled with love, faith, and God's blessings.

As we embark on the chapters ahead, remember that this book is just the beginning. Fatherhood is a lifelong journey that will continually evolve and deepen. It is my prayer that this book serves as a valuable resource for you in these initial stages and that it lays the groundwork for a rich, faith-filled experience as a father.

1

A Miracle Begins

Understanding the wonder of conception is the first step in taking on the role of a father. It is a biological miracle intricately woven into the heavenly fabric of creation. This chapter begins with an examination of the scientific conception process, followed by a discussion of how this process reflects the amazing creation of God.

The moment a woman's egg and a man's sperm meet is known as conception. This connection, which frequently occurs in the fallopian tube, signifies the start of a new life. It's a methodical and exquisitely designed procedure. After leaving the ovary, the egg descends the fallopian tube and may come into contact with a sperm cell there. Fertilization takes place if a sperm enters the egg and is successful. The zygote, or newly formed cell, then starts to travel toward the uterus while rapidly dividing and developing.

It's crucial for fathers to comprehend this process. It not only readies you for your part in this journey, but it also helps you appreciate the fine intricacies of life's beginnings. This process's meticulous attention to detail at each stage is proof of the complex architecture of human life.

This biological process is more than merely a sequence of cellular occurrences, according to Christian doctrine. It is an illustration of God's creative ability and proof of His presence in the very fabric of existence. Psalm 139:13–14 in the Bible states, "For you wove me together in my mother's womb; you created my inmost being. I thank you for making me fearfully and wonderfully. These lines eloquently capture the awe and respect that ought to accompany the conception process.

This extraordinary incident offers you a chance to consider God's role as the Creator as you consider it. He is directly involved in the genesis of life, not just a bystander. His divine purpose is the source of this new being's every cell, heartbeat, and breath. This knowledge should astound you and instill a strong sense of duty in you as you get ready to become a father. You are involved in a heavenly act of creation, not merely a biological procedure.

This is a great opportunity to ponder and pray during this stage of pregnancy. It's crucial to turn to God in prayer as you and your companion set out on this adventure, asking for His blessings and direction. Offer up prayers for the mother's well-being and the safety of the unborn child. As you get ready to care for and raise this child in accordance with His will, seek His wisdom.

It's also a good moment to consider how you fit into this adventure. Think about the various ways you may assist your partner on a spiritual, emotional, and physical level. Consider the alterations taking place and how they align with your religious beliefs. You have the chance to strengthen your bond with God and ready your heart for the trip that lies ahead.

The first step to becoming a father is to understand conception. It's an ideal place to start for your future journey because it combines science with spirituality. Let the wonder of life's beginning serve as a daily reminder of God's love, strength, and design for your family as you go through this month.

Praying For Your Growing Family

As you enter this new stage of your life, prayer becomes a vital resource for supporting your expanding family. It's crucial to turn to God in these early stages of pregnancy with prayers for protection, wisdom, and thankfulness. Let's look at several ways you might utilize prayer to uplift and guard your family spiritually at this critical time.

Start your prayers with gratitude. Acknowledge the gift of fresh life that God has given to you and your companion. Thank God for this bounty and acknowledge each kid as a special creation of His. "Behold, children are a heritage from the Lord, the fruit of the womb a reward," declares Psalm 127:3. Thank God in your prayers for this blessing and the chance to become a parent.

Pregnancy's early phases can be a period of excitement and wonder as well as worry and fear. It's normal to be concerned for your partner's and your unborn child's safety and well-being. Pray to God about these worries. Seek His hand to keep your family safe. Offer prayers for your partner's health and well-being as well as the baby's. Philippians 4:6-7 reminds us to "let your requests be made known to God in everything by prayer and supplication with thanksgiving," so keep that in mind.

You might be nervous about what lies ahead as a soon-to-be father. Now is the time to ask God for insight and direction. Ask God to grant you the capacity to be a loving partner during the pregnancy. Pray for discernment while making choices, for endurance under pressure, and for fortitude to meet the difficulties that lie ahead. James 1:5 exhorts us to seek wisdom from God, who gives freely to everyone without pointing out their shortcomings.

Try to get your partner to join you in prayer. During this period of transition, your partnership can be strengthened and mutual support can be given by this shared spiritual practice. When you pray together, you become closer to God and to each other by sharing your hopes, anxieties, and thankfulness. Matthew 18:20 tells us that "I am with them wherever two or three come together in my name."

Considering the wonder of life from a scriptural viewpoint can bring consolation and understanding. The Bible is full of verses that describe God's hand at work in creation and His concern for all human existence. Scriptures like Jeremiah 1:5, "I knew you before I formed you in the womb," serve as a constant reminder of God's intimate knowledge of and purpose for each and every life. These contemplations help strengthen your understanding of the miracle growing inside your partner's womb and your responsibility to protect and care for this unborn child.

Early pregnancy is a period for personal spiritual development as well. Think back on your relationship with God as you offer prayers for your family. Think about the ways in which becoming a father could bring you closer to God. During this period, study texts about fatherhood and the family and develop your knowledge of God's role in your life and the life of your household.

Let prayer be your constant companion during the first month of your pregnancy. You can express your thanks, ask for protection and direction, and deepen your relationship with God and your partner by praying. In addition to supporting your expanding family, this practice will get your heart ready for the adventure that comes with becoming a father.

We explore the rich tapestry of biblical reflections that honor God's hand in creation and the beginning of life in this last portion of Chapter 1. As you begin the path of parenthood, these reflections provide profound understanding and motivation, serving as a constant reminder of the divine essence of the developing life.

Reflections On The Miracle of Life

In this final section of Chapter 1, we examine the rich tapestry of biblical comments that acknowledge God's hand at work in creation and the beginning of life. These reflections serve as a constant reminder of the divine essence of the developing life, offering profound understanding and motivation as you embark on the path of motherhood.

Numerous texts in the Bible uphold the sanctity and value of life, particularly that of a child. Psalm 139:13–16 contains one of the most moving passages, discussing God's close involvement in the development of life in the womb. This verse encourages you to acknowledge God's hand at every stage of your child's development and to marvel at the miraculous process of life's beginnings.

It's critical to understand God's sovereignty as you consider these biblical passages. This fundamental tenet of the Christian faith recognizes that God is in charge of all facets of human existence, including the process of conception. "I am the Lord, the maker of all things, who stretches out the heavens and spreads out the earth by myself," declares Isaiah 44:24. This verse affirms God's role in the miracle of your child's life and serves as a reminder of His ultimate authority over creation.

The Bible frequently refers to parenthood as a blessing and a gift. Children are described as a heritage and a reward from the Lord in Psalm 127:3-5. Ponder these verses and the blessings and burdens that come with being a parent. This viewpoint has the power to alter your perception of the path ahead, helping you to perceive it as a spiritual journey that God has entrusted to you rather than just a sequence of physical changes.

There may be times when becoming a father brings with it uncertainty and anxiety. A potent strategy for navigating these feelings is to look to Scripture for solace and encouragement. You can find inspiration in Philippians 4:13, "I can do all things through Christ who strengthens me," which serves as a reminder that you are not traveling alone. You have access to God's strength, which will provide you courage and support as you get ready to become a father.

One recurrent subject in the Bible is God's purpose and design for our life. This fact is addressed in Jeremiah 29:11, "For I know the plans I have for you, declares the Lord, plans for welfare and not for evil, to give you a future and a hope." It's consoling to know that God has a purpose for your family while you and your spouse wait for the birth of your child. This plan shapes your child's life and your position as a parent, not just for the here and now but also for the future.

During the first month of your pregnancy, immerse yourself in Scripture and use this time to be ready to be a father. The Bible gives parents insight and direction by outlining guidelines for raising kids in a way that pleases God. For example, Ephesians 6:4 counsels fathers to discipline and train their children in the ways of the Lord. By thinking about these verses, you can lay the groundwork for becoming the kind of father you want to be.

As you come to the end of this first chapter, consider the wonder of life and God's involvement in it. As you start this journey, use the biblical reflections to be your guide and source of consolation. Remind yourself that you are a part of something amazing and heavenly as a father. Accept this responsibility with love, faith, and the knowledge that God is always at your side.

Journey of the Heart - Devotional

In the stillness of your heart, as you stand at the dawn of fatherhood, let's embrace a journey that intertwines the wonder of life's beginning with the profound truths of faith. This path of fatherhood is not just a biological venture; it's a spiritual odyssey, interwoven with the miraculous and the divine.

Understanding the genesis of life, the miraculous conception process, is your first step into fatherhood. Each moment of this journey, where a new life is being woven together in the womb, is a testament to the awe-inspiring work of God. As Psalm 139:13-14 reminds us, every cell, every heartbeat of your unborn child, is a part of God's masterful creation, a living testimony to His intricate design and unfathomable love.

As you walk this path, let prayer be your steadfast companion. In the quiet moments, lift your heart in gratitude to God for the gift of new life He has entrusted to you and your partner. Recognize this child as a divine heritage, a blessing as proclaimed in Psalm 127:3. In the early stages of this journey, where excitement and apprehension may intertwine, turn your worries into prayers. Philippians 4:6-7 teaches us to bring everything to God in prayer, enveloping our requests in thankfulness, a practice that brings a peace that surpasses all understanding.

Your role as a father-to-be may bring a myriad of emotions and questions. In these moments, seek wisdom and guidance in your prayers. Ask God to equip you with the strength to support your partner, the discernment to make wise decisions, and the fortitude to embrace the challenges ahead, as encouraged in James 1:5. In this journey of parenthood, you are not alone; God's wisdom and strength are a prayer away.

This journey also offers a beautiful opportunity to strengthen your bond with your partner through shared prayer. As Matthew 18:20 reminds us, where two or three gather in His name, there He is with them. Praying together can deepen your connection with each other and with God, sharing hopes, fears, and gratitude.

Remember, as you embark on this journey, that you are part of something far greater than just a biological process. You are participating in a divine act of creation, shaping a life that is fearfully and wonderfully made. Embrace this calling with love, faith, and the assurance that God is with you every step of the way, guiding, strengthening, and blessing you as you step into the sacred role of a father.

I humbly ask for Your guidance and strength. Bless my partner and our unborn child, keeping them safe and healthy. Fill my heart with love, patience, and wisdom to be the father You call me to be. Amen.

2

Seeing God's Hand

Greetings from the second month of this amazing adventure. This is the month that your baby experiences some of the earliest and most important developmental milestones as their small life inside the womb expands. It's a time when God's exquisite creation and skillful design are wonderfully displayed. Let's examine these changes and consider their spiritual implications.

Your baby changes dramatically in the second month of pregnancy. The primary organs start to form at this stage. The heart beats more regularly now than when it was just a slight flutter. The brain, spinal cord, and other essential organs have their foundations set. Little buds begin to form that will eventually become arms and legs. It's a time of tremendous expansion and development, demonstrating the intricacy and beauty of God's work.

It might be inspiring for a soon-to-be father to see these improvements, even in an indirect way. It is a chance to be in awe of the wonder of life, which is so finely woven and perfectly arranged by God. Even though they are minute and invisible, each of these changes brings us one step closer to the creation of a novel, distinct person—a being made in God's image (Genesis 1:27).

Your baby's heart is developing this month, and that's one of the biggest changes. This critical organ, so necessary to life, starts to beat and take shape. The heart is frequently used in the Bible as a metaphor for life and the core of our existence. "Above all else, guard your heart, for everything you do flows from it," Proverbs 4:23 reminds us. Imagine your baby's heart starting to beat and consider how important it is to nurture both bodily and spiritual existence.

Additionally, the physical form of your baby began to take shape this month. The small buds that develop into limbs are a blatant example of God's meticulous labor. It's amazing to consider how these little beginnings will grow into feet that can walk, hands that can hold objects, and a mouth that can talk. According to Psalm 139:15–16, "When I was woven together in the depths of the earth, my frame was not hidden from you when I was made in the secret place." Your eyes beheld my undeveloped body. As you consider your child's physical development, you might use this verse as a meditation to be reminded of the love and care that God gives to all of His creations.

It's a good idea for you as the father to consider how you will be supporting this new life when these physical changes take place. You are invited to actively participate in the nurturing and care of this kid, just as God is deeply concerned in the development of this child. This engagement extends to creating a caring, safe, and spiritually nurturing environment in addition to meeting bodily requirements. Fathers are urged by Ephesians 6:4 to raise their kids according to the rules and guidance of the Lord. This teaching starts even before your child is born, as you get your home and heart ready for their arrival.

Continue to be your partner's advocate throughout this month by offering practical assistance and prayer. Offer up prayers for your partner's health and strength, as well as for your baby's continuous healthy development. Provide practical assistance by going to prenatal appointments, assisting with everyday chores, or just being there to offer emotional support.

Pause for a moment to consider the remarkable advancements that have occurred. Every turn on this trip is evidence of God's amazing plan and His tender touch in the creation of life. Allow this insight to strengthen your faith and resolve to be the greatest father you can be—a parent who embodies God's compassion, support, and direction.

Faith and Patience in Early Pregnancy

Although your baby undergoes significant physical changes in the second month of pregnancy, these changes are frequently invisible to the untrained eye. As you wait for obvious evidence of the new life developing within your partner, you must have a strong sense of faith and patience during this stage. Let's discuss the value of patience and trust in these early, frequently unclear phases of pregnancy.

Pregnancy's early phases are a time of invisible miracles. Even though the kid is not yet visible or palpable, amazing growth and development are taking place inside the womb. This time frame serves as a lovely metaphor for faith—believing in things we cannot see. Faith is described as "assurance about what we do not see and confidence in what we hope for" in Hebrews 11:1. Adopting this faith as a soon-to-be father entails believing in God's purpose for your developing child, even when it isn't yet apparent.

Christian virtue of patience is highly regarded, and it is especially important during the early stages of pregnancy. "Let perseverance finish its work so that you may be mature and complete, lacking nothing," states James 1:4. Patience in this period involves active trust in God's timing rather than passive waiting. It's realizing that every developmental stage of your child, no matter how tiny or invisible, is important and occurs in accordance with God's exquisite plan.

Your spouse may experience fear and uncertainty throughout the early stages of pregnancy. During this time, your understanding and patience are greatly appreciated. Recognize that your spouse is going through major emotional and physical changes and offer support and empathy in response. Provide solace, pay attention to her worries, and stand by her side. She may get a great deal of comfort and security from your patience and collected manner.

When uncertainty and lack of patience become overwhelming, resort to prayer. An effective strategy for finding strength and serenity is prayer. Bring to God your worries, aspirations, and hopes for your family. Philippians 4:6-7 exhorts us to give gratitude and offer our petitions to God in prayer instead of worrying. Allow the incomprehensible peace of God to keep your hearts and thoughts safe in Christ Jesus.

Pregnancy's second month offers a chance to accept God's timing. This phase serves as a gentle reminder that everything happens at its set time, despite the intensity of your want to see and touch your baby. "There is a time for everything, and a season for every activity under the heavens," according to Ecclesiastes 3:1. Considering this verse, accept the season you are in and remember that every phase of life has a purpose and beauty of its own.

Together with your partner, use this time to deepen your religion. Discuss your aspirations for your child, pray aloud, and share scriptures. By strengthening your relationship and expanding your family's religion, this common spiritual journey can provide a solid foundation for your future.

Growing in faith, accepting God's timing, and having faith are lessons that you will apply to your role as a parent as well as being a part of the pregnancy experience. As you prepare for the amazing journey that lies ahead as a parent, let these early stages of pregnancy deepen your faith and patience.

Scriptural Insights on Creation and Life

Now let us look to the scriptural truths that highlight the beauty and holiness of life, particularly when it is developing in the womb. These revelations not only give you a better understanding of the physiological changes your kid is going through, but they also give this amazing process a spiritual context.

The Bible starts with the creation myth, in which God's omnipotence and inventiveness give rise to life in all its forms. "So God created mankind in his own image, in the image of God he created them; male and female he created them," reads Genesis 1:27. As your child grows, consider this verse. It alludes to the fundamental reality that everyone is a reflection of God, including your unborn child. This insight gives you a newfound sense of wonder and accountability in your duty as a father. Not only are you seeing a new life form, but you are also seeing the emergence of a being created in the image of its Creator.

Scripture values life highly and accords it great dignity. "Before I formed you in the womb I knew you, before you were born I set you apart," declares Jeremiah 1:5. This scripture implies that every individual has a distinct identity and purpose in God's eyes even before birth. Take into account the amazing idea that God has already prepared a plan and purpose for this new existence as you see your developing child. This knowledge can help you appreciate the experience of being pregnant even more and raise expectations for the special person your child will grow up to be.

With all of its developmental milestones, the second month of pregnancy is a tribute to the miracle of life's beginnings. Particularly pertinent are Psalm 139:13–14, where the singer acknowledges God's role in forming his deepest being. You are encouraged to marvel at the complex process of development taking place inside the womb by this chapter. It's an exhortation to recognize and be grateful for the delicate, heavenly work that these formative years of life are enacting.

It's crucial to acknowledge God as both the Creator and the Sustainer of life as your child grows and matures. "Because in him we live and move and have our being," says Acts 17:28. This verse serves as a reminder that God sustains life at every breath, heartbeat, and instant. It's a reassurance that God is actively involved in creating and maintaining this new life in the context of your baby's development.

Make thoughtful use of these biblical precepts for contemplation and preparation in prayer. Offer up prayers for your partner's health and well-being as well as for your child's continuing growth and development. Allow these verses to direct your prayers, bringing thanksgiving, amazement, and hope for the life being woven together inside your womb.

Lastly, think about how you fit into God's plan for your family as you ponder these verses. For your child, you have the responsibility of being a provider, guardian, and spiritual guide. Early in pregnancy is a great moment to renew your commitment to these tasks and ask God to give you the discernment, fortitude, and direction you'll need to be a father.

Think for a moment on the profound insights into the genesis and development of life that are found in the Bible. These formative years for your child are more than just biological benchmarks; they are a part of a heavenly masterpiece that God himself has crafted. Allow these realizations to arouse astonishment and thankfulness in you and equip you for the upcoming adventure of parenthood, which is based in faith and directed by God's kind hand.

Embracing the Miracle - Devotional

This period marks some of the earliest and most significant developmental milestones in your baby's life, a time when the wonder of God's creation and His masterful design are magnificently displayed. As a father-to-be, witnessing these changes, albeit indirectly, offers a profound opportunity to marvel at the miracle of life, so intricately woven and perfectly orchestrated by God. Each minute, unseen change draws us closer to meeting a unique individual, crafted in God's image (Genesis 1:27).

This month, your baby's heart begins its vital rhythm, transitioning from a faint flutter to a regular beat. This organ, so essential to life, embodies the biblical metaphor for life's core (Proverbs 4:23). As you reflect on your baby's heartbeat, consider the importance of nurturing both physical and spiritual life. Simultaneously, the physical form of your baby takes shape - limbs start as tiny buds, destined to become arms and legs, symbolizing God's meticulous work (Psalm 139:15-16). This development invites you, as the father, to ponder your role in nurturing this new life, shaping a caring, secure, and spiritually nurturing environment, as advised in Ephesians 6:4.

Support your partner through this journey with practical help and prayer. Pray for her health and strength, and for your baby's continued healthy growth. Your engagement is not just physical but deeply spiritual as well.

Now, let's turn to faith and patience, virtues essential in the early, often unseen stages of pregnancy. This period is a beautiful metaphor for faith - the belief in what we cannot see, as described in Hebrews 11:1. Patience is equally important, as expressed in James 1:4, signifying an active trust in God's timing. Embrace this time as a lesson in trusting God's plan and supporting your partner through her emotional and physical transformations. Prayer becomes a refuge in moments of uncertainty (Philippians 4:6-7), offering strength and peace.

The second month of pregnancy is an opportunity to embrace God's timing, a reminder that every moment unfolds in its divinely appointed time (Ecclesiastes 3:1). Use this time to deepen your faith with your partner, fostering a strong spiritual foundation for your family.

Lord, I thank You for the gift of new life growing within my family. Guide me to be a supportive, loving, and faithful partner and father. Bless my partner and our baby with health and strength. Fill our hearts with patience, trust, and peace as we embark on this journey together. Amen.

3

Faith Takes Shape

The growth inside the womb accelerates as you approach the third month of this incredible adventure. The passage from the embryonic to the fetal stage is a critical developmental milestone for your unborn child. This is a time for in-depth spiritual contemplation since your baby's physical changes can reveal important truths about the nature of God's creation and the development of your faith.

Your unborn child, now known as a fetus, begins to rapidly develop in the third month. The organs develop more and begin to work. The bones start to stiffen, facial features become more pronounced, and fingers and toes are clearly delineated. During this stage, the fetus begins to resemble a human being, making the miracle of life even more apparent.

This is truly an amazing turnaround. It brings to mind the Psalmist's statement, "I praise you because I am fearfully and wonderfully made," found in Psalm 139:14. Think about the meticulous attention to detail God has put into each and every one of creation as you evaluate these changes. Every growing organ and every tiny finger is evidence of His exquisite labor.

This developmental stage of the fetus can be compared to the process of spiritual formation. Our faith must expand and grow, just as the fetus grows and develops to prepare for life beyond the womb. In 1 Corinthians 3:2, the apostle Paul discusses transitioning from spiritual milk to solid food. As you embark on your road to become a father, think about how your own faith is growing. Exist any facets of your spiritual life that require more development or maturation? Now is a great moment to look for a closer relationship with God and a greater understanding of him.

The fetus's distinct identity changes along with its development. Even at this early age, every infant is unique in their features and traits. This individuality is a lovely illustration of how God makes every person special and has a purpose for them. This is reminded of in Jeremiah 29:11, when God announces His intentions to provide us with a future and hope. While you wait for your baby to arrive, consider the special place they will hold in the world and the special parenting adventure you will embark on.

Pregnancy might still be unpredictable throughout the third month. Many parents wait for the second-trimester ultrasound to see their unborn child in order to feel a stronger bond. Similar to Abraham's faith in Hebrews 11:1, who trusted in God's promises even if they were not yet apparent, this time requires faith. As a soon-to-be father, accept this waiting time with faith and have confidence in God's plan for your family and kid.

Keep praying for your partner's health and the development of your child. In addition to being consoling, these prayers uphold your position as your family's spiritual head. As you get ready to welcome this new life into your world, pray for discernment and direction. Additionally, pray for your own spiritual development so that you might fulfill God's calling to be a father.

As the fetus develops, so too should your perception of your paternal role. Now is the moment to consider how you will support your child's spiritual development. Parents are encouraged to teach their children about God's rules and to have daily conversations about them, according to Deuteronomy 6:6-7. Start thinking about how you will raise your child in a home that fosters spiritual development and how you will share your beliefs with them.

Trusting in God"s Plan

Many things about the pregnant experience are still unclear and unknown, particularly in the third month. This is a great moment in the journey to concentrate on having faith in God's plan for your family's future as well as for the growth of your infant. Let's explore the significance of this trust and how it can influence your impending fatherhood.

Pregnancy frequently carries with it a mixture of excitement and anxiety throughout the third month. Even though there has been a lot of development, many of the changes are not readily apparent, and it may take some time for the reality of becoming a parent to set in. Your faith can provide you with comfort and strength during these uncertain times. "Trust in the Lord with all your heart and lean not on your own understanding; in all your ways submit to Him, and He will make your paths straight," is what Proverbs 3:5–6 exhorts us on. This verse serves as a potent reminder to trust God's knowledge and purpose even in the face of uncertainty.

The idea that God ultimately has authority over the universe and our lives is known as the sovereignty of God, and it is one of the major tenets of Christian faith. This idea can provide a great deal of comfort during pregnancy, which is an uncertain time. Keep in mind that "in all things God works for the good of those who love him, who have been called according to his purpose" (Romans 8:28). This assurance, which serves as a constant reminder that God is in charge of everything on this path with love and purpose, can help allay fears and anxieties.

An essential instrument for developing faith in God is prayer. Ask questions, voice your anxieties, and share your hopes in prayer. Offer up prayers for your partner's health and well-being, your child's growth and wellbeing, and your own readiness to become a father. You can give God your problems through prayer and find comfort in His promises. Keep in mind Philippians 4:6-7, which states that if you give thanks to God for everything you ask for, God will grant you peace and keep your hearts and minds in Christ Jesus.

As you move through the third month of your pregnancy, make the most of this opportunity to trustingly become ready for motherhood. Beyond just the pragmatics, this preparedness also entails a spiritual readiness. Think about how you can make your home a reflection of your faith in God. Consider the principles and teachings you wish to teach your child—principles that are based in faith and dependence on God.

Your partner might be feeling uneasy and worried at this time as well. Offer her encouragement and support while standing by her side in faith. Read verses in the Bible that attest to God's omnipotence and concern. Your common religious beliefs can deepen your relationship and give your expanding family a strong basis.

Prayers For Health and Safety

It is important to emphasize the importance of prayer in obtaining health and safety for the mother and the developing child as we now concentrate on the major changes that occur at the end of the third month of pregnancy. This last section provides suggestions on certain prayers and spiritual activities that might help your family thrive.

For the woman, the third month of pregnancy may be a period of physical and mental change. It's a time when more attention and assistance are frequently needed. Your well-wishes for your partner's health and resilience are greatly appreciated as a soon-to-be father. Please offer up prayers for her physical health so that she won't have any pain or difficulties. Additionally, offer up prayers for her emotional and mental well-being so that she can go through this life-changing period in peace and joy. As the Bible instructs us to "bear one another's burdens" (Galatians 6:2), you are helping your partner by praying for them.

This is a crucial and delicate month for your baby's growth. It's a time to offer prayers focused on the fetus's healthy development and progress. Offer up prayers for the healthy development of every organ, strong bones, and appropriate production of every physical characteristic. These prayers can be guided by Psalm 139:13–16, which gives a stunning example of God's involvement in the complex process of creating life in the womb. Recall that you are asking God to watch over and provide for your child through your prayers.

Ask God for wisdom and direction to help you navigate the journey ahead, in addition to prayers for health and safety. Ask God for wisdom as you make decisions about your pregnancy and the things you need to prepare for your new family member. Ask God to give you insight into becoming the father He desires you to be and wisdom on how to help your partner most effectively. James 1:5 tells us to ask God, who gives freely to everyone without finding fault, if we lack insight.

Make time to pray with your partner, if at all possible. This communal spiritual activity can be a very powerful means of fostering relationships with God and one another. It can improve your bond, foster understanding between you, and forge a spiritual connection that will support your family. Jesus states, "Where two or three gather in my name, there I am with them," in Matthew 18:20. This assurance highlights the need of praying as a pair.

Your prayers at this time are starting a legacy of faith that you are creating for your family, not simply for the here and now. You are creating the groundwork for a household where faith is paramount by making prayer and spiritual development a priority right now. One of the best gifts you can give your child is this legacy.

Trusting in God's Guiding Hand - Devotional

As you traverse the miraculous path of fatherhood, especially in these early months of pregnancy, you are witnessing firsthand the awe-inspiring process of life unfolding. This journey, marked by growth, faith, and trust in God's plan, is not only about the physical development of your unborn child but also about your own spiritual maturation as a father-to-be.

In the third month, your child transitions from an embryo to a fetus, a significant milestone mirroring the deepening of your own faith journey. As you marvel at the rapid development of your child's tiny organs, bones, and features, remember the words of the Psalmist in Psalm 139:14, "I praise you because I am fearfully and wonderfully made." Each intricate detail of your child's formation is a testament to God's meticulous craftsmanship and a reflection of His love and care in creation.

This period of fetal growth resonates deeply with the process of spiritual formation. Just as your child is preparing for life beyond the womb, your faith too is being nurtured and developed for the new life ahead as a father. In 1 Corinthians 3:2, Paul speaks of moving from milk to solid food in our spiritual journey. Contemplate on this: Are there areas in your faith needing further growth or maturity? Embrace this season as an opportunity to seek a deeper relationship with God and a better understanding of His will for you and your growing family.

Your child, unique even at this early stage, symbolizes the individuality and purpose God bestows upon each of us. Jeremiah 29:11 reminds us of God's plans to give us hope and a future.

Reflect on the unique role your child will play in the world and the special journey of parenting that lies ahead for you.

During this time of waiting and uncertainty, much like Abraham's faith in Hebrews 11:1, embrace faith in God's promises. Pray for your partner's health and your child's development, reaffirming your role as the spiritual leader of your family. These prayers are not just petitions for wellbeing but are foundations of your growing relationship with God as you prepare to welcome this new life.

As your child's physical form takes shape, so too should your vision of fatherhood. Consider how you will guide your child's spiritual growth, taking inspiration from Deuteronomy 6:6-7, which urges parents to impart God's commandments to their children. Begin to envision a home environment where faith flourishes and where God's teachings are a daily conversation.

Entering the third month of pregnancy often brings a blend of excitement and uncertainty. This is a crucial time to lean on your faith and trust in God's plan, as emphasized in Proverbs 3:5-6. This period is a powerful reminder of God's sovereignty, a central tenet of Christian belief, providing comfort and reassurance as stated in Romans 8:28.

Prayer becomes a vital tool during this journey. Use it to express your concerns, hopes, and gratitude. Philippians 4:6-7 encourages us to bring our requests to God with thanksgiving, assuring us of His peace. Pray for your partner, your child, and your preparedness for fatherhood. These prayers are not only a source of comfort but also a means of surrendering your anxieties to God and embracing His peace.

Support and encourage your partner, sharing scriptures that affirm God's power and care. This shared faith will strengthen your bond and lay a solid foundation for your growing family.

Heavenly Father, guide us in love and wisdom as we nurture this new life and grow in faith together. Amen.

4

Breath of Life

The development of your unborn child's respiratory system marks a significant milestone as you enter the fourth month of your pregnancy. This important stage represents a spiritual link to life's breath, a gift from God, as well as a physiological advancement. We examine this significant advancement and its more profound spiritual ramifications in this part.

Your baby's lungs are growing quickly in the fourth month, getting ready for their first breath after birth. The fetus starts to breathe even though its lungs are still developing. This breathing preparation is a vital stage in your baby's development and is necessary for life beyond the womb.

This is a very interesting discovery from a biological standpoint. It involves the lungs' complex structural creation, which gets them ready to oxygenate blood after birth. As a soon-to-be father, you can gain a greater understanding of the intricacy and wonder of human existence by indirectly observing this aspect of growth.

The Bible frequently uses breath as a metaphor for spirit and life. "Then the Lord God formed a man from the dust of the ground and breathed the breath of life into his nostrils, and the man became a living being," according to Genesis 2:7. This verse eloquently captures the essence of God's breath. As your child learns to breathe, take some time to consider the amazing gift of life.

The breath of life also serves as a reminder of the Holy Spirit, who is frequently represented in the Bible as wind or breath. The source of all vitality, life, and energy is the Spirit. When you reflect on your child's growth, remember that this new life is not only a physical expression but also a spiritual one, imbued with God's breath.

You should concentrate your prayers this month on your baby's respiratory system's good development. Please offer up prayers for the right formation of the lungs and for the smooth completion of all breathing-related processes. These prayers are expressions of faith in God's plan and provision for your child, in addition to wishes for physical well-being.

You have a life-giving and nurturing role in your child's development as a parent. The process by which your infant learns to breathe can be compared to how you contribute to the spiritual and emotional growth of your child. Consider how you may provide an atmosphere that supports your child's spiritual and emotional growth in addition to their physical health. Think on the lessons, principles, and values you wish to impart; these are what will give them meaning and vitality.

Supporting Her Through Love and Prayer

Your spouse may suffer more noticeable physical and mental changes as the fourth month of pregnancy goes on. As a soon-to-be father, this is a crucial time for you to actively support your partner. Let's explore how you can show your partner support, adoration, and understanding during this crucial time by providing love and prayer.

The fourth month may bring about a number of changes for your companion. She might begin to manifest more physically, and as the reality of her approaching motherhood sinks in, she might experience a spectrum of emotions on an emotional level. It is imperative that you exhibit empathy, comprehension, and patience throughout this period. Learn about these changes so that you can better understand her needs and emotions.

Empathic listening is one of the most effective ways you can help your spouse. This entails paying attention to her worries, pleasures, and anxieties without attempting to solve issues or provide answers right away. Sometimes, just being there, listening, and validating her feelings is the most consoling thing you can do.

You and your partner can find a great deal of solace and strength in prayer. Offer up prayers for her well-being, the baby's health, and mental clarity. Praying with your partner is another way you may uplift and assist her. Your relationship can be strengthened and you can both receive spiritual and emotional support from this shared spiritual practice. Recall that Philippians 4:6 instructs us to "let your requests be made known to God in everything by prayer and supplication with thanksgiving, and do not be anxious about anything."

Apart from providing psychological and spiritual assistance, providing useful assistance can be immensely advantageous. This could include taking care of her everyday tasks, going with her to prenatal visits, or just making sure she gets enough time to rest and take care of herself. Being of service in small ways is a great way to show someone you care and support them.

It's essential to have a loving and supportive environment at home. This encompasses both the interior and exterior spaces as well as the mood. Think before you speak and behave. By telling your spouse that she is strong and capable of being a mother-to-be, you can support and encourage her.

Take advantage of this opportunity to be ready for your baby's arrival as a couple. Talk about your goals and strategies for becoming parents, as well as how you can help one another in this new position. This planning involves more than just making the necessary arrangements; it also involves coordinating your goals and expectations as parents.

Understanding the Growth Spurt Through Faith

It's critical to acknowledge the notable physical growth surge your child is going through and comprehend how, as an expectant father, this matches your own spiritual development. Together, we will examine the similarities and differences between your baby's physical growth and your own spiritual journey, offering advice and understanding that will enhance your experience throughout this life-changing period.

In the fourth month of pregnancy, your baby experiences a significant growth surge. The baby's health depends on this quick physical development, which also gets them ready for life outside the womb. In a similar vein, you are going through a stage of spiritual development as a soon-to-be father. You are expected to develop spiritually with your child, expanding your knowledge of faith, parenthood, and your place in the family, in the same way that your child does physically.

Your baby's growth spurt might be compared to the obstacles and chances for personal development you encounter on your spiritual path. You must grow spiritually in order to properly lead and care for your family, just as the infant needs to grow physically in order to survive and prosper. This could entail conquering obstacles in your life, reassessing your priorities, and strengthening your connection with God.

Growth involves major changes in both the physical and spiritual realms. Faith and confidence in God's plan are necessary for accepting these changes. Faith is defined as "assurance about what we do not see and confidence in what we hope for," according to Hebrews 11:1. Allow your observation of your child's invisible development to strengthen your belief in the invisible work God is performing in your own life.

An essential tool throughout this growing season is prayer. For your baby's ongoing healthy development, offer up prayers. Pray for your own spiritual development at the same time. Pray to God for discernment, endurance, and compassion as you get ready to become a father. Ask Him for advice on how to be a devoted, godly parent who shows your child how much He loves them.

There are many lessons to be learned throughout the growing process for both you and your infant. Every developmental milestone your baby reaches represents a step closer to adulthood and independence. You see every obstacle and shift as a chance to develop your faith and character. Accept these teachings, for they are preparing you for the duties and rewards of becoming a father.

During this period of rapid growth, consider the legacy of religion you are leaving for your child. Your personal spiritual development also lays the groundwork for the spiritual development of your family. Think about the principles, behaviors, and values you wish to impart in your child and begin implementing them in your daily life right away.

Embracing the Breath of Life - Devotional

As you enter the fourth month of your pregnancy, witnessing the development of your unborn child's respiratory system, you are not just observing a milestone in physical growth but also experiencing a profound spiritual journey. This critical stage in your baby's development—preparing for their first breath—is a miraculous blend of God's handiwork and biological wonder. In these moments, you stand at the intersection of life's breath, a divine gift, and a testament to the marvels of human life.

Reflecting on Genesis 2:7, where God breathes life into man, you realize the profound symbolism of breath in your faith. As your child's lungs prepare for their first breath, it's an opportunity to ponder the extraordinary gift of life, a life infused with the Holy Spirit, the ultimate source of vitality and energy. This period isn't merely about physical growth but a spiritual awakening, recognizing your child as not just a physical being but a soul cherished by God.

Your role as a father extends beyond providing for physical needs. As your baby learns to breathe, consider how you can nurture their spiritual and emotional well-being. Contemplate the values and lessons you want to impart, understanding that these will be the breath of life that sustains them in their spiritual journey.

Your devotion extends to your spouse, too, as she endures significant physical and emotional changes. This phase requires your empathy, understanding, and unwavering support. Empathetic listening becomes a sanctuary for her, where her feelings are acknowledged and respected. Engage in prayer together, seeking comfort and guidance from God, as Philippians 4:6 suggests. Your practical support in daily tasks and emotional encouragement are vital in creating a nurturing environment for your growing family.

Heavenly Father, bless our growing child with health and breath, guide us in love and faith, and strengthen our family in Your grace. Amen.

5

Over Halfway There!

A crucial turning point in your pregnancy experience occurs at the fifth month, when the gender of your unborn child is frequently revealed. This discovery provides a meaningful chance to celebrate the uniqueness of God's design for every life, not merely a joyful milestone. Let's examine this revelation's relevance and how it can help you comprehend and appreciate God's creative brilliance on a deeper level.

Finding out their baby's gender is a happy and exciting occasion for many expectant parents. It can be a joyful moment, signaling the start of a new chapter in the pregnant journey. This realization frequently gives the pregnancy a more "real" sense and enables you to begin picturing a more tangible future with your child. It's a chance to develop a closer bond with your child by envisioning their future selves.

God's hand is at work in this intricate biological process that determines your baby's gender. It serves as a reminder of how meticulous and intricate His effort was in producing a new life. According to Psalm 139:13–16, we are fearfully and wonderfully created, knit together in our mother's womb. Finding out the gender of your child is a concrete manifestation of this reality and evidence of how special God made each and every one of us.

Finding out your child's gender can also be an opportunity to consider the uniqueness and purpose that God has for each of us. "Before I formed you in the womb I knew you, before you were born I set you apart," declares Jeremiah 1:5. This scripture emphasizes that God knows and loves your child, regardless of gender, and that they have a special purpose and life path. This discovery can be both sobering and inspiring for parents, as you consider the part you will play in raising and developing this special person.

You may find yourself reflecting more on how to raise your child now that you know your baby's gender. Think about how raising a son or daughter in the modern society entails teaching them faith, love, and respect. Regardless of gender, consider how you might support your child in accepting and understanding who they are in Christ.

Make use of this opportunity to offer up prayers for your child's future. Offer up prayers for their well-being, moral fiber, and connection to God. Seek insight and direction so that you can raise children in accordance with God's plan. Additionally, offer up prayers for your spouse and yourself so that you can be the kind of parents your child needs—people who can help them in all facets of their lives.

As you gain more insight into your child's identity, embrace the journey ahead with love and faith. This gender revelation is about recognizing and becoming ready for the special person whom God is entrusting to your care, not only about blue or pink, trucks or dolls.

Sensory Development

The level of your baby's sensory development is unprecedented. In addition to being a crucial time for your unborn child's physical development, this phase serves as a moving parallel for your own spiritual development as an anticipating father. Let's examine the amazing advancements in your baby's senses and how your own spiritual development can be reflected and inspired by them.

Your baby's sensory development changes significantly in the fifth month. The baby's ears have grown to the point that they can distinguish noises, such as the calming beat of the mother's heart and even muted sounds from the outside world. The baby's ability to feel is also developing, as it begins to investigate its own body and environment inside the womb. These advancements set the groundwork for future learning and interactions and represent a significant stage in the baby's connection with its surroundings.

Your own spiritual awareness can be compared to how your baby's senses are developing. As your child starts reacting to outside stimuli, you may also notice that you are become more aware of the spiritual side of life and parenting. This may show itself as an increased capacity for empathy, a better comprehension of your religion, or a closer bond with your personal spiritual principles.

As your infant's world grows in all directions, think about how you are answering the invitation to grow spiritually. Are you paying closer attention to what your religion has to teach? Are you planning for your child's needs and growing more attuned to your partner's needs? Similar to how a baby develops their senses, you have the chance to touch, feel, and explore your faith in new and deeper ways at this time.

Use introspection and prayer to foster this spiritual development. Seek out times of reflection and solitude so that you might hear from God. Examine texts that discuss the joys and duties of parenthood. Allow the development of your baby's senses to encourage you to become more deeply aware of and knowledgeable of spirituality.

Your baby's learning and comprehension of the world come before their sensory development. In a similar vein, this period of spiritual development equips you to mentor your child spiritually. Think about how you will model Christian values for your child, how you will introduce faith to them, and how you will create a home where spiritual discovery is encouraged.

Scriptural Encouragement for the Halfway Point

Midway through your pregnancy is a big deal, and it's a good idea to take a minute to stop, think, and read Scripture for inspiration. The purpose of this part is to support your faith and fortitude while you await the birth of your child by offering biblical guidance and encouragement during the second half of your pregnancy.

It's time to celebrate reaching halfway and express gratitude for the journey thus far. The Bible makes frequent mention of being thankful in every situation. "Give thanks in all circumstances; for this is God's will for you in Christ Jesus," reads 1 Thessalonians 5:18. Consider the gifts you have experienced during the first five months, both large and small. Take this opportunity to thank God for all of the blessings you have already received, including protection and advancement, as well as the joy and optimism that the future brings.

There could be additional difficulties and unknowns throughout the second half of the pregnancy. It is imperative to keep in mind and derive strength from God's faithfulness. Consider Lamentations 3:22–23, which states, "Great is your faithfulness; the steadfast love of the Lord never ceases; his mercies never come to an end; they are new every morning." These verses serve as a reassuring reminder that God will continue to lead and provide for you and your family, just as He has done thus far.

Pregnancy is a journey that requires both trust and anticipation. "Trust in the Lord with all your heart and lean not on your own understanding; in all your ways submit to Him, and He will make your paths straight," is what Proverbs 3:5–6 exhorts us on. This trust will be essential to you as you move through the upcoming months, overcoming any obstacles along the way and getting ready for the arrival of your kid. Keep in mind that God has a great plan for your family and that He is by your side at all times.

For the rest of the pregnancy, patience and wisdom will be needed for both the birth plan and the adjustment to being a parent. If anybody among you lacks wisdom, James 1:5 advises to ask God, who freely gives to everyone without finding fault, and it will be given to you. Utilize this pledge to ask God for guidance when making decisions and taking action. Furthermore, practice patience by realizing that each stage of this journey is a part of God's impeccable timing.

Get your heart ready for fatherhood as you anticipate meeting your child. Fathers are advised to "bring them up in the discipline and instruction of the Lord" (Ephesians 6:4). Think about how you can bring up your child in a way that pleases God and fosters a love for Him. This preparation establishes the foundation for a godly legacy and is not only practical but also spiritual.

A Journey of Faith and Love - Devotional

As you stand at the threshold of fatherhood, the revelation of your unborn child's gender at five months is a profound moment, marking not just a joyful milestone, but a deeper understanding of God's magnificent creation. This discovery is a vivid reminder of the unique purpose God has for each of us. It's a moment that brings the reality of your upcoming role as a father into sharper focus, inviting you to begin dreaming and planning for a future filled with nurturing and guiding this precious life.

This pivotal point in your journey is echoed in the words of Psalm 139:13–16, where the intricate craftsmanship of God in forming life is celebrated Knowing your child's gender not only personalizes this journey but also brings to life the scripture in Jeremiah 1:5, which speaks of God's intimate knowledge and unique plan for every individual. As a father, this realization is both humbling and exhilarating, igniting a sense of responsibility and wonder at the role you will play in shaping this new life.

In understanding your child's gender, you're invited to ponder upon the ways to raise them in today's world. Teaching them faith, love, and respect transcends gender norms. It's about instilling in them a strong sense of identity in Christ. This period is an opportunity to deepen your prayers, seeking wisdom and guidance to fulfill God's vision for your family. Pray for your child's future, their moral integrity, and their relationship with

God. Pray, too, for the strength and insight to be the parent your child needs.

As you delve into understanding your child, embrace this journey with a heart full of faith and love. This is more than a revelation of gender; it's about preparing to welcome and nurture the unique individual God is entrusting to your care.

Parallel to the physical development of your child is the amazing progression of their sensory abilities, which offers a poignant analogy for your spiritual growth as a father-to-be. Your baby's increasing sensitivity to sounds and touch in the womb is a mirror to your expanding spiritual awareness and connection. This phase is a call for introspection and growth, urging you to explore your faith more profoundly and prepare spiritually for parenthood.

Dear Lord, guide me in fatherhood, bless my child with health and happiness, and let us grow in Your love and wisdom together. Amen.

6

A Leap of Viability

Since it frequently signifies the point of viability, the beginning of the sixth month of pregnancy is a significant event. This indicates that, with medical help, the baby has a possibility of surviving outside the womb if it is born at this point. This noteworthy developmental milestone for your child serves as both a medical and a spiritual reminder of the value of having faith in God's perfect timing.

The word "viability" denotes a significant developmental milestone for your child: their lungs are maturing and they are getting stronger every day. This development is evidence of the wonder of life and the complex plan by which God created the human form. When the baby reaches this point, it emphasizes their growing independence and resilience, which fills many expectant parents with a mixture of relief, appreciation, and wonder.

The idea of viability and the Christian doctrine of faith in God's timing mesh wonderfully. "There is a time for everything, and a season for every activity under the heavens," according to Ecclesiastes 3:1. This verse exhorts us to acknowledge and honor the divine timing in all facets of life, including your child's growth and development. As you celebrate this accomplishment, think about how you may keep trusting God's plan for your pregnancy and the future of your unborn child.

You get to experience the wonder of growth and development as you marvel at your baby's progress to reach this stage of viability. The time frame serves as a striking reminder of Psalm 139:14, which says, "I praise you because I am fearfully and wonderfully made." Every developmental stage of your unborn child is a mirror of God's complex plan and handiwork.

As viability approaches, your prayers may become more profound. Offer up prayers for your baby's overall wellbeing, their essential organs' continuing strength, and their continued health and growth. Additionally, when your girlfriend approaches the last trimester, keep praying for her health and fortitude. By saying these prayers, you can put your family's journey in God's capable hands.

When a situation reaches the stage of viability, it's also time to start getting ready for the potential of becoming parents sooner rather than later. This is a spiritual as well as practical preparation. In addition to assembling baby necessities and arranging the nursery, think about how you will provide your child with a loving, spiritually-filled atmosphere. Start imagining the spiritual legacy you want to leave behind.

This period serves as a potent reminder of how fleeting life is and how much responsibility you have been given as a parent. With hope and expectation, look forward to the upcoming months, prepared to take on the joys and challenges that lie ahead.

Preparing Spiritually for Parenthood

During the sixth month of pregnancy, when viability is reached, you should also be strengthening your spiritual preparation for motherhood. This time allows you to consider how you will raise and train your child spiritually as well as physically and emotionally. Let's explore how you can get ready for the holy duty of raising a kid in the faith.

One of your main responsibilities as a soon-to-be father will be to lead your family spiritually. To do this, one must develop a heart that looks to God for insight and direction. Seek guidance from God on how to guide your family by spending time in prayer and reading the Bible. "Train up a child in the way he should go; even when he is old he will not depart from it," says Proverbs 22:6. Think back on this verse and what it means to raise and mentor your child in their religion.

Becoming a parent spiritually requires creating a household where faith is appreciated and carried out. Think about how you can make biblical teaching, prayer, and worship a regular part of your family's routine. This could entail establishing or enhancing your own routines, such family Bible study time, regular devotions, or prayer before meals. The intention is to create a house that both reflects and fosters a relationship with God.

Youngsters pick up a lot of knowledge from the adults in their lives. Your attitudes, words, and deeds will have a big impact on how your child understands faith. Make it your goal to live a life that exemplifies love, grace, and integrity—a godly example. We are urged to "be imitators of God, as beloved children" in Ephesians 5:1-2. And follow Christ's example of love, whereby he offered his life for us. Consider how you, as a father, can set an example of these Christ-like traits.

Joining a faith community can offer resources, encouragement, and support when you start your parenting journey. Seek out a community where your family can experience spiritual growth if you're not currently actively participating in a church or faith-based organization. These relationships can provide your child and you with important direction, companionship, and a sense of belonging.

Being a parent involves more than simply meeting your child's physical and emotional needs; it also involves assisting them on their spiritual path. Take some time to consider how you will explain your faith, impart biblical principles, and address any spiritual queries your child may have as they get older. As you get ready to lead your child, be willing to grow and learn about your own beliefs.

This preparation is about preparing your heart and house to be a place where faith is cultivated and lived out, not merely about making physical arrangements. Accept this period of preparation and have faith that God will provide you with all you need to tackle the wonderful and difficult task of raising a child in the faith.

Preparing Your Home for Fatherhood - Devotional

Embracing the Journey: Preparing Your Heart and Home for Spiritual Parenthood

In the tender moments of the sixth month of pregnancy, as you witness the marvel of viability, your heart is drawn into a profound reflection on the journey ahead. This significant milestone marks not just a medical triumph but a spiritual awakening, a reminder of God's perfect timing in every breath of life.

The concept of viability, where your child's lungs mature and strength burgeons, is a testament to the intricate design of our Creator. In these moments, as you marvel at this tiny being's resilience, you're reminded of the awe-inspiring nature of life itself, woven meticulously by God. Psalm 139:14 echoes in your heart, "I praise you because I am fearfully and wonderfully made." Your child, even in the womb, is a living portrait of God's intricate handiwork and love.

As parents-to-be, your journey intertwines with the Christian doctrine of faith in God's timing. Ecclesiastes 3:1 whispers a timeless truth, "There is a time for everything, and a season for every activity under the heavens." This verse is not just a soothing balm but a call to action, inviting you to lean into the divine rhythm of life, embracing each stage of your child's development with trust and grace.

In this sacred time, your prayers deepen, encompassing the wellbeing of your growing baby and the health of your partner entering the final trimester. These prayers are more than words; they are acts of surrender, entrusting your family's journey to God's capable hands.

Preparing for parenthood transcends the physical realm, entering a spiritual domain. It's a time to lay the foundation of a home that radiates love and faith, a sanctuary where your child will learn about God's love, grace, and truth. Imagine the spiritual legacy you wish to impart, a legacy that will guide your child long after they step into the world.

Remember, your role as a father is pivotal in shaping this spiritual journey. Proverbs 22:6 guides you, "Train up a child in the way he should go; even when he is old he will not depart from it." This wisdom calls you to lead by example, nurturing a home where prayer, worship, and biblical teachings are the bedrock of everyday life.

Lord, guide us in raising our child with love, wisdom, and faith, reflecting Your grace and nurturing a heart devoted to Your path. Amen.

7

Smiles of Hope

You are getting closer to the time when you will meet your baby as you approach the seventh month of pregnancy. This is often a special period of yearning mixed with happiness and excitement. Your religion as a soon-to-be parent can greatly enrich this experience by turning the waiting into a time of joyful anticipation and spiritual growth.

One of the most important stages of the pregnancy experience is the third trimester. This is the moment when the reality of soon becoming a parent really sinks in. This understanding causes a mixture of joy and anxiety in many people. Your faith can provide you courage and consolation during these trying times. Consider the advice given to us in Romans 12:12 to "Be joyful in hope, patient in affliction, faithful in prayer." As you traverse the intricacies and emotions of the third trimester, let this passage serve as a guide for your mindset.

As the time for your child's birth approaches, give yourself permission to experience the excitement and wonder of waiting. Picture yourself holding your infant for the first time, seeing their face for the first time, and hearing their screams for the first time. These ideas can evoke great happiness and a deep sense of thankfulness to God for the gift of life. As we are reminded in Psalm 127:3, "Offspring are a reward from the Lord, children are a heritage from him." While you wait for your reward—your child—enjoy this moment.

Make the most of this time of waiting to strengthen your connection with God. Take some time to pray and meditate, asking God to give you wisdom and direction for the path ahead. This is a spiritual prelude to parenthood, a lifelong journey, not simply a birth. Pray to God to fill your heart with the love, endurance, and discernment that a father needs, as well as to prepare you for the trials and changes that lie ahead.

You can use this period of waiting to talk to your partner about your spiritual journey. Talk about the aspirations you have for your child and how your faith affects them. Please share scriptural references and prayers that have held special value for you at this time. This mutual spiritual experience can deepen your couple's bond and bring you together in a shared future vision for your family.

It is crucial to have faith in God's timing as the weeks and days lead up to the birth of your child. Every pregnancy and delivery are different, and things don't always go according to plan. Putting your faith in God's perfect time will help you feel less anxious and keep your attention on the excitement of the impending birth. Isaiah 55:8 nudges us to put our faith in God's flawless plan by reminding us that His ways and ideas are higher than ours.

Allow your faith to enrich this experience by bringing hope and tranquility into it. This last trimester is a unique opportunity to spiritually get ready for the amazing path of parenthood that lies ahead, not merely a countdown to delivery.

Reflecting on the Development of Life

As your baby's development reaches new heights, it's a time to be in wonder and contemplate. This stage of pregnancy brings to light the amazing beauty and intricacy of life, which is a gift from God. Comprehending and valuing these advancements will strengthen your bond with the wonder developing inside your partner's womb and heighten your sense of thankfulness and obligation as a prospective parent.

Your baby's brain is growing quickly at this point as it gets ready to leave the womb. The baby's senses are developing, and they can now react to touch, light, and sound more clearly. Your unborn child may now react to your voice or a light touch on your partner's stomach, allowing for a closer bond between you and the child.

These complex changes serve as a striking reminder of Psalm 139:14, where the Psalmist extols himself, saying, "I am fearfully and wonderfully made." As you consider the development of your child, consider this verse: every new growth is evidence of the intricate and amazing job that God did in creating a new life.

Think about the spiritual aspect of life's gift as you watch these advances. Life is a priceless gift from God, full of possibility and meaning, not just a biological process. Your baby's every motion and heartbeat serve as a constant reminder of this priceless entrustment placed in your capable hands. "Every good and perfect gift is from above, coming down from the Father of the heavenly lights," as James 1:17 reminds us. Accept this moment as a chance to celebrate the amazing gift of life that God has given you.

The duty to care for life arises from the recognition of it as a divine gift. This duty involves fostering your child's spiritual and emotional growth in addition to giving them physical care and safety. Think about the ways you will provide an atmosphere in which your child can develop love, wisdom, and faith. Start praying for wisdom on how to help your child develop these attributes.

This is a special time in your pregnancy to bond with your unborn kid. Spend time conversing and singing with your child, as well as involving yourself at times when you can feel their movements. These exchanges bolster your relationship with your child and your participation as an active participant in their life journey.

Use this time to get ready while maintaining optimism and faith in God's plan for the birth. Anxieties about giving birth and being a parent can coexist with the excitement of finally meeting your child. Rely on your faith for assurance and serenity. Philippians 4:6-7 exhorts us to give thanks to God and to submit our requests without worry. Have faith that He will give you the courage and discernment you require for childbirth and beyond.

The seventh month is when a pregnancy enters its last stages. This is the time to enjoy every second of it while you wait for the baby to arrive. Treasure the relationship you have with your partner and your child, and keep your house and heart ready for the newest member of your family.

Think back for a moment on the profound bonds that were forged during this time: bonds with God, your partner, and your unborn child. During this time, you should prepare your heart and soul for the transformative role of fatherhood in addition as physically. Enjoy the present moment and look forward to the pleasures and difficulties that lie ahead. Do it with thankfulness, hope, and trust.

Nurturing Your Relationship with God and Family

It's a great time to concentrate on strengthening your ties with God and your family as the seventh month of pregnancy progresses. These connections are the backbone of your support network and will be vital to the development of your new child. Insights and advice on strengthening these vital ties throughout this critical stage of the journey are provided in this section.

The cornerstone of your spiritual life is your relationship with God, which has a big impact on how you view fatherhood. Make greater use of this time for meditation, prayer, and reading the Bible. Take part in spiritually energizing activities, including going to church, joining a Bible study, or taking quiet time to spend in nature. We are urged to "Be still, and know that I am God" in Psalm 46:10. Take some time to be still so you can hear what God could be saying to you about being a parent.

A new baby's arrival is a momentous occasion for the whole family. In order to create a caring and supportive family environment, this time is essential. Include your other children in the baby's preparations if you have any, as this will help them embrace and comprehend their new role as older siblings. To ensure that your relationship stays healthy and robust, make time for your mate. "Be completely humble and gentle; be patient, bearing with one another in love," is what Ephesians 4:2–3 counsels. Do everything in your power to maintain the bond of peace and the unity of the Spirit. Use these ideas to improve the relationships in your family.

Having honest and open communication is essential to keeping partnerships strong. Invite family members to share their opinions, feelings, and hopes for the new child. Pay close attention, offer comfort and encouragement, and reassure. This routine will not only help the family acclimate to the changes a new baby brings, but it will also set the stage for continuous, honest communication.

A potent tool for fostering family unity and welcoming God into your house is prayer. Make it a habit to pray together, maybe before bed or during mealtime. Your family's faith can be strengthened by these times of group prayer, which can also offer consolation and direction as you all get ready for the new member.

A couple's relationship may undergo substantial alterations as a result of parenthood. Talk to your partner about your goals, worries, and expectations for parenting during this time. Together, ask God for direction and pray for discernment and fortitude to meet the difficulties and rewards of parenthood. Honor your voyage as a joint enterprise, deepening your alliance in the process.

Think about the kind of religious legacy you want to leave for your family as you get ready for your baby to arrive. Consider the customs, beliefs, and values you want to leave behind. Leaving a lasting legacy involves more than just educating your child about religion; it also involves leading an example of values and beliefs. "Blessed are his children after him who walk in integrity," according to Proverbs 20:7. For your family, try to live up to this verse.

These connections form the cornerstone of your child's upbringing and will influence how they view religion, love, and society. Seize this opportunity to build a loving, open-minded, and religious family atmosphere as you get ready for the next phase of your life that will begin with the birth of your kid.

God's Gift is Right Around the Corner - Devotional

In this final trimester, let the words of Romans 12:12 resonate within you: "Be joyful in hope, patient in affliction, faithful in prayer." This time is a testament to the beauty of creation and the strength of your faith. Embrace the emotions, knowing that each one is a step towards becoming a parent, a role ordained and blessed by God. As Psalm 127:3 reminds us, children are indeed a heritage from the Lord, a reward that enriches your life in immeasurable ways.

This period is an opportunity to strengthen your connection with God, seeking His guidance and wisdom. Parenthood is a lifelong journey that starts long before the birth of your child. Pray for love, endurance, and discernment, qualities essential for a father. Share this spiritual journey with your partner, discussing your aspirations and the role of faith in your growing family. These conversations can deepen your bond and align your vision for your family's future.

As you navigate the uncertainties and joys of this period, remember Isaiah 55:8. God's plan is perfect, even when it diverges from our expectations. Trust in His timing and let this faith bring peace and focus to your experience.

Reflect on the development of your baby, a marvelous display of God's craftsmanship. Each milestone in their growth is a testament to the wonder of life, as described in Psalm 139:14. This is a time to acknowledge the gift of life as more than a biological process, but a divine entrustment, as James 1:17 points out. Each heartbeat of your child is a reminder of the responsibility and privilege you have as a parent.

Consider the emotional and spiritual growth of your child as well. Think about how you will create an environment where love, wisdom, and faith can flourish. Engage with your unborn child, talking and singing to them, feeling their movements. This interaction builds a bond that transcends the physical realm.

Lord, grant us strength, wisdom, and joy as we embrace parenthood.
Bless our growing family with love, faith, and unity in Your grace.
Amen.

8

Nearing the Promise

As you enter the eighth month of pregnancy, a crucial stage in your unborn child's growth is reached. The majority of their organs are now completely formed and getting ready to function outside the womb. This amazing advance in your baby's growth is not only a physical milestone but also evidence of the wonders of God's creation.

By the eighth month, important things start to happen. Your baby's lungs are nearly fully developed and ready for that first vital breath after birth, but their brain is still developing quickly. The liver can now process certain waste products, and the kidneys are operating at maximum capacity. Your baby is virtually ready for life beyond the mother sanctuary based on all these changes.

Thinking back on these advancements can be really encouraging. It's a potent illustration of Psalm 139:14, where the Psalmist declares, "I praise you, for I am fearfully and wonderfully made." Every developmental stage that your unborn child experiences in the womb is a manifestation of God's exquisite and skillful handiwork.

The eighth month is a time to celebrate life's miracles and acknowledge God's hand at work in every aspect of your baby's growth. Every part of your baby's development, from the way each organ forms to the intricate wiring of the brain, is evidence of the divine artistry. It's a chance to grow in your faith and understanding of the sacredness of life.

It's crucial to keep praying for your baby's organs' health and correct operation while they finish developing. Offer up prayers for the brain and lungs in particular, as these are essential for life and growth outside the womb. By confirming your faith in God's providence and protection, you can dedicate your child's health and destiny to His care through these prayers.

During the last phases of your pregnancy, you should also start preparing yourself spiritually and mentally for the birth. In addition to knowing how a delivery occurs, this preparation entails strengthening your spiritual foundation in anticipation of the transformative experience of being a parent. Take some time to pray, asking God to give you courage, tolerance, and discernment.

Seek His comfort and serenity to allay any worries or anxiety around the impending birth.

This is a critical time to deepen your relationship with your spouse by supporting and understanding her through the mental and physical strain of the last few weeks of pregnancy. Be there, pay attention, and offer assistance. Attend prenatal visits and talk about birth plans to share the experience and make sure you are both ready and on the same page for what lies ahead.

This is a time to celebrate your baby's developmental milestones, grow in your spiritual readiness, and fortify your family's increasing unity. Anticipate with optimism and delight the day you will at last lay eyes on your child.

Understanding the Final Preparations

The eighth month of pregnancy is a critical time for both spiritual and physiological preparations. This is the time when your baby's growth is at its peak and major birth preparations are being made. You can move through this period with confidence and faith if you understand these latter stages from both viewpoints.

In terms of medicine, your baby undergoes significant development throughout the eighth month to be ready for life outside the womb. The developing baby's brain keeps growing quickly, honing the connections that will enable cognitive and sensory processing. The lungs are almost fully developed and ready for that crucial first breath following birth. In addition, the baby starts to assume the birthing position, usually lowering its head toward the birth canal.

Prenatal checkups and heightened surveillance occur in tandem with these bodily changes. It is crucial to evaluate the baby's position, growth, and general health at these appointments, as well as your partner's preparedness for giving birth. During these visits, topics like as the birth plan, possible labor indicators, and pain relief choices may be discussed.

The eighth month is a time to grow in your spirituality and put your trust in God's plan for your family. It's a time to take stock of your journey thus far and to eagerly anticipate the birth of your child. With the words, "The Lord will keep you from all harm— he will watch over your life; the Lord will watch over your coming and going both now and forevermore," Psalm 121:7-8 provides consolation and assurance. As you get ready for the birth, let this scripture be a source of comfort and strength.

You still need to include prayer in your spiritual preparations. Continue to pray for your partner's health and strength, for a safe and easy delivery, and for the wellbeing of your unborn child. By putting your trust in God, you can ask for His protection and direction through these prayers.

As your child's delivery draws near, set aside some time to emotionally prepare yourself for the life-changing experience of parenthood. Think about the kind of father you want to be and the characteristics of a home where faith is a stronghold. Think about the spiritual heritage you want to leave your child and how you will help them to comprehend and accept their faith.

Finally, the last few weeks before giving birth are an important time to fortify your marriage. Keep lines of communication open with your spouse and talk about any worries you may have about being a parent and having a child. Recognize and acknowledge your partner's physical and emotional changes while providing emotional support and understanding. As you both assume the roles of father and mother, this unity and support are essential.

Now is the moment to get involved with your religion community. Talk to your small group or church family about your hopes and requests for prayer. Your community's encouragement and support can be very helpful, providing a feeling of mutual hope and faith.

During this time, you should focus on establishing your connections, building your spiritual life, and being ready to welcome your kid into a loving, religious home in addition to making sure you are medically prepared. With confidence, anticipate the birth, knowing that God's presence will lead you every step of the way.

Biblical Perspectives on the Final Stage

It's enlightening to consult the Bible for viewpoints and anecdotes that provide consolation and direction as you near the end of month eight and consider the last phases of pregnancy. These biblical ideas will help you comprehend your trip and the amazing event that will occur at its conclusion on a deeper level.

Having faith in God's plan even in the face of uncertainty is one of the most important truths the Bible imparts. The tale of Abraham and Sarah, who endured years of childlessness, is a prime example of persistent confidence in God's promises. Their narrative, which can be found in Genesis chapters 17–21, serves as evidence for the conviction that, despite their occasional deviation from our own expectations, God's designs are always ideal. Let your child's narrative encourage you to have faith in God's impeccable timing and plan for your family while you wait for their birth.

The Bible is filled with accounts of people who, in the face of uncertainty, found strength in God. Think about Joshua's journey, wherein he guided the Israelites into the Promised Land. God gives Joshua 1:9 encouragement, saying, "Be strong and courageous." The Lord, your God, will be with you wherever you go, so do not be afraid or give up. This scripture can be a potent reminder that God is giving you strength and bravery throughout these last stages of pregnancy.

One of the Bible's main themes is the effectiveness of prayer. Philippians 4:6-7 exhorts us to give gratitude and offer our petitions to God in prayer rather than worrying. Throughout these last few weeks, let prayer be your haven. Offer up prayers for a smooth and safe birth, for your spouse and child's health, and for your own courage as you adjust to becoming a father. In addition to asking God for assistance, prayer can help one discover comfort and serenity in His company.

The arrival of a kid signifies the start of a new chapter in your life as well as the epic tale that God is crafting for your family. Your child has a specific position in God's plan, just as every biblical character has a distinct part to play in His greater story. Examine Jeremiah 29:11, which gives us assurance about God's intentions to provide us with a future and hope. Accept the impending birth as the beginning of this thrilling new journey.

Being a parent demands love and humility, two traits that Jesus demonstrated throughout His life. Little children are greeted and blessed by Jesus in Mark 10:14–16, demonstrating the significance of children in God's Kingdom. Aim to resemble Christ in all that you do as you get ready to receive your child: love, humility, and hospitality.

Lastly, rejoice in the pleasure and happiness of a new life. We are reminded that "offspring are a reward from him, and children are a heritage from the Lord" in Psalm 127:3. Let this fact fill your heart with appreciation and excitement as the birth of your child draws near. A lovely reminder of God's love and faithfulness is the birth of a new life.

The biblical viewpoints and tales presented here are not merely timeless literary works, but also dynamic expressions that provide direction, solace, and resilience. Allow them to uplift and equip you for the exquisite and hallowed process of bringing a new life into the world—a spiritual as well as a physical journey.

Embracing the Divine Journey - Devotional

In the quiet of the eighth month, as you watch over the gentle rise and fall of your spouse's belly, you are participating in a divine journey. A journey marked not just by the growth of your unborn child, but by the deepening of your faith and the strengthening of your family bond. This period is a tangible reminder of God's intricate design and His profound involvement in our lives.

At this stage, your baby, a wonderful creation of God, is reaching significant milestones. Their organs, nearly fully developed, are ready to function outside the womb. Such progress mirrors the words of Psalm 139:14, "I praise you, for I am fearfully and wonderfully made." Each kick and movement beneath your spouse's heart is a testament to God's exquisite craftsmanship.

This time serves as a call to celebrate life's miracles and to recognize God's hand in every tiny detail of your baby's development. The intricate wiring of the brain, the near-complete development of the lungs—every aspect is a stroke of divine artistry. It's an opportunity to grow in awe and understanding of the sacredness of life.

In these final weeks, your prayers become even more crucial. Pray for the health and proper functioning of your baby's organs, especially the brain and lungs, which are vital for life outside the womb. Such prayers reaffirm your trust in God's providence and your dedication of your child's health and future to His care.

But your journey is not just about watching and waiting. It's about preparing—spiritually and mentally—for the transformative experience of fatherhood. Pray for strength, wisdom, and patience. Ask God to guide you in nurturing and leading this new life He has entrusted to you.

This period also calls for deepening the bond with your spouse. Be present, both physically and emotionally. Share in the anticipation and the planning. This unity and mutual support are crucial as you step into the roles of mother and father.

Reflecting on Biblical Perspectives, think of Abraham and Sarah, whose story in Genesis is a beacon of faith in God's perfect timing. Or Joshua, who was reminded to be strong and courageous, for God was with him wherever he went (Joshua 1:9). These narratives are not just ancient texts; they are reminders of the constancy of God's presence and the power of faith.

In the final stages, let prayer be your refuge. Philippians 4:6-7 encourages us not to be anxious but to present our requests to God. Pray for your partner, your coming child, and for your own heart as it prepares to embrace a new life.

Remember, the arrival of your child marks the beginning of a new chapter in the grand story God is weaving for your family.

Jeremiah 29:11 assures us of God's plans for hope and a future. Embrace this new chapter with joy and expectation.

Heavenly Father, lead us in this journey of parenthood. Bless our child's health, strengthen our bond, and fill our hearts with Your love and wisdom. Amen.

9

The Final Countdown

You are on the verge of a significant life transition as you begin your ninth and last month of pregnancy. This time, which is frequently characterized by a mixture of excitement and anxiety, necessitates embracing patience, faith, and confidence in God's plan. It's a time to take stock of your journey so far and get ready for your child's arrival on an emotional and spiritual level.

The amazing journey of pregnancy comes to an end in the ninth month. It's a period when excitement is at its height and the reality of becoming a parent approaches quickly. Your baby is physically positioning itself, gaining weight, and completing the last stages of labor. This month is about accepting the last phases of this life-changing adventure with faith and trust in God's perfect timing, for you as a soon-to-be father.

When the deadline draws near, it's normal to experience anxiety or impatience. But now is the perfect moment to put your faith and confidence in God's plan in action. Comfort and strength are provided by Isaiah 40:31, which states, "But those who hope in the Lord will renew their strength." They will fly like eagles, run without tiring, and stroll without losing consciousness. This verse can serve as a helpful reminder of the power that comes from putting your faith in God, particularly when you're waiting or facing uncertainty.

It is also a time for spiritual preparation throughout the last month. Develop a closer relationship with God in prayer, asking for insight and direction for the impending birth and the journey of motherhood. Pray for your ability to be a supporting presence during the birth process, as well as for your partner's and your child's health and safety during the delivery. Recall that prayer is an expression of faith in God's care and provision as much as a request for assistance.

Consider your emotional preparedness in addition to your spiritual preparation. Think about the adjustments that becoming a father will bring about and how you will accept these new duties. Being emotionally prepared is essential because it will enable you to provide good support for your partner and form a bond with your child from the time of birth. Children are described as a blessing and a reward from the Lord in Psalms 127:3-5. Allow this viewpoint to influence how you handle the pleasures and difficulties of becoming a father.

In the final weeks, your spouse will probably be going through a mix of emotions and physical discomforts. Be a constant source of encouragement, providing consolation, empathy, and useful assistance. Keep up with prenatal visits, assist with the last-minute baby preparations, and make sure your spouse feels cherished and supported. Wives are to be loved like Christ loved the church, according to Ephesians 5:25. During these final weeks, let your actions be guided by this call to unselfish love.

Spend some time cherishing these final moments of pregnancy, even though the excitement of meeting your kid might often be overwhelming. Think back on the journey you've taken with your partner and the personal development you've both undergone. Honor your partner's fortitude and resiliency and thank them for strengthening your relationship during this difficult period.

This is a time to strengthen your faith in God, be ready mentally and spiritually to become a parent, and show your partner patience and love. Anticipate your child's arrival with great anticipation, prepared to embrace this new member of your family.

Preparing For Birth

As the ninth month progresses, getting ready for birth becomes a spiritual journey rather than just a practical arrangement. This preparation entails having confidence in God, realizing the sanctity of childbirth, and putting your trust in him. Let's talk about how to become spiritually ready for your baby's arrival and turn this event into a life-changing spiritual adventure.

Deep faith in God is necessary during the birthing process because of its inherent difficulties and unpredictable nature. This confidence is about more than just having faith that everything will work out the way it is supposed to; it is also about finding comfort in the assurance that God is in charge, no matter what. "Trust in the Lord with all your heart and lean not on your own understanding; in all your ways submit to Him, and He will make your paths straight," is what Proverbs 3:5–6 exhorts us on. Use this knowledge as you get ready for the birth, having faith that God will lead you and your spouse every step of the way.

There may be a lot of emotional and physical intensity during the last few weeks of pregnancy and the actual delivery. It is imperative that you draw strength from your faith throughout this period. Prayer on a regular basis, scripture meditation, and group worship can give strength and consolation. Take Hannah's account from 1 Samuel 1, where she confided in God to satisfy her greatest desire for a child. Her unwavering faith and steadfast prayer life are encouraging examples of asking God for help when things get tough.

The act of creating a new life is a holy undertaking. It's a chance to personally experience the wonder of creation that God has given to us. Consider the sacredness of this procedure and how it ties you and your spouse into the divinely intended cycle of life. As you approach the birth, Psalm 139:13–16, where the psalmist acknowledges God's hand in his creation, can inspire and awe you.

It's critical that you play the supportive partner role during labor and delivery. Get ready to provide others spiritual and emotional support. This could be providing a comforting presence, encouraging words, and praying with and for your partner throughout labor. Recognize that your assistance is essential to the birthing process and that it reflects God's love and concern.

The excitement grows closer to the actual birth. Now is the moment to concentrate on the amazing trip that will soon come to an end when you meet your child. Let us pray for a safe and healthy delivery and express our gratitude during this time of waiting. Keep in mind that every moment of this journey brings you one step closer to experiencing the miracle of newly discovered life, which is a blessing from God.

Make the most of this opportunity to strengthen your bond with your partner and your unborn kid. Share your aspirations for your child's future in conversation with them. Tell your girlfriend how much you care and assure her that you will be there for her on the trip ahead. These ties will not only improve your relationship but also establish a lasting bond that will benefit your child.

Allow your faith to serve as the cornerstone of these arrangements, directing you to put your faith in God, draw strength from His presence, and recognize the majesty of childbirth. With a heart full of faith, hope, and love, prepare yourself for the arrival of your child and welcome this new life into a world that represents God's goodness and concern.

Trusting in God's Perfect Timing

Trusting in God's perfect timing for the birth and unfolding of new life is a crucial topic to embrace as you navigate these last days of the ninth month. This confidence is essential because one of the few unknown components of pregnancy is often the time of childbirth. By accepting this uncertainty with trust, we can turn these last days into a time of spiritual growth and submission to God's will.

By its very nature, childbirth is unpredictable. Even with the best-laid intentions, a baby's actual birth date and method may differ. Although this uncertainty can be unsettling, it also offers a chance to develop a strong faith in God. Go back to Proverbs 16:9: "Humans plot their course in their hearts, but the Lord determines their steps." This verse serves as a reminder that, although we can arrange things, God ultimately controls the path things take, even when your child is born.

Letting up of the need to oversee every detail of the birthing process is a necessary part of yielding to God's purpose. It entails having faith that God's love and presence will always be present, regardless of how the birth turns out. Consider the life of Jesus' mother, Mary. As demonstrated in Luke 1:38, "I am the Lord's servant...," she responded to the uncertainties and difficulties she faced with confidence and surrender to God's plan. May you fulfill your promise to me.

During these last days, ask for patience and serenity in your prayers. Pray for God to ease your worries and to fill your heart with an unfathomable serenity. Ask God to grant you the serenity and confidence to welcome the birth process in whatever form it takes. The peace of God, which surpasses human comprehension and envelops our hearts and minds in Christ Jesus, is mentioned in Philippians 4:7. Allow this calm to serve as your solace and protector.

It's crucial to support your partner during this waiting period. She can be feeling tired, uncomfortable, and worried about the birth herself. Provide consolation, confidence, and encouragement. Your assistance can keep her composed and in control, fostering a happy atmosphere while you both wait for your child to arrive.

Finally, cherish these last seconds before taking the life-changing journey into parenting. Take this time to consider your journey thus far, your personal progress, and the changes that lie ahead. Savor these final moments spent with your spouse, as they signify the close of one chapter and the start of a new one in your family's history.

Allow God's love and perfect timing for the impending arrival of a new life to fill your heart. Pregnancy is an amazing combination of physical, emotional, and spiritual experiences that culminate in this crucial moment of birth. With an open heart and a spirit tuned to God's guidance and love, embrace the last countdown.

March Towards the Final Arrival - Devotional

As the final month of pregnancy dawns, it brings with it a symphony of emotions. The crescendo of anticipation, coupled with waves of uncertainty, marks a time of profound transition. You, standing on the precipice of fatherhood, are about to embark on a journey that intertwines patience, faith, and an unwavering trust in God's plan. This devotional is your companion in these transformative days, seeking to deepen your connection with the Divine and prepare your heart for the wonders of parenthood.

In the ninth month, life seems suspended in a moment of divine creation. Your baby, growing and positioning for birth, symbolizes the culmination of God's miraculous handiwork. It is in these days that faith takes center stage. Isaiah 40:31 reminds us, "But those who hope in the Lord will renew their strength." Let this verse be your anchor, providing solace and strength as you navigate the uncharted waters of fatherhood.

This period calls for spiritual fortitude. Engage in prayer, seeking God's wisdom and guidance for the journey ahead. Pray for strength, for your partner, and the safe arrival of your child. Remember, prayer is as much an act of faith as it is a request for divine intervention. Emotionally, prepare to embrace the shifts that fatherhood brings. The Psalmist's words, "Children are a heritage from the Lord" (Psalms 127:3-5), should frame your perspective, viewing fatherhood not just as a responsibility, but as a divine blessing.

Your role as a supportive partner is pivotal. Offer comfort, empathy, and practical help, embodying Christ's love for the church (Ephesians 5:25). This love is selfless, patient, and kind, qualities essential in these final weeks. Reflect on your journey together, honoring the resilience and strength of your partner and the bond that has deepened through this shared experience.

As you prepare for birth, understand that this is more than a physical process; it is a spiritual journey. Trust in God's plan is paramount. Proverbs 3:5-6 guides us to "Trust in the Lord with all your heart," a reminder to rely on God's wisdom and guidance. Draw strength from your faith, find inspiration in the stories of the Bible, like Hannah's unwavering prayer in 1 Samuel 1, and marvel at the sacred act of creating life, as expressed in Psalm 139:13-16.

Dear Lord, grant us strength, patience, and love as we welcome this new life. Bless our family with Your guidance and everlasting grace. Amen.

10

A New Begining

Upon welcoming your child into the world, the period immediately following birth, known as the "tenth month," can be a transformational experience. This new chapter in your family's history is being written, and it is a moment filled with much love, joy, and spiritual importance. Let's examine the intricacies of this fresh start and the part your faith plays in embracing and raising your child.

The moment your child is born is one of unmatched wonder and delight. It's the result of months of waiting and a physical representation of life's wonder. Experiences like your child's first cry, first touch, and first look into their eyes can often leave a lasting impression on you. According to Psalm 127:3, "Offspring are a reward from Him, and children are a heritage from the

LORD." Acknowledge this as a priceless gift from God, a just recompense for putting your faith and confidence in His hands during your pregnancy.

Your responsibilities as a Christian parent expand with the birth of your child. This responsibility includes fostering your child's spiritual development in addition to caring for and safeguarding them. As you caress your infant, remember that you have been given the duty of bringing him up in God's love and wisdom. Fathers are advised to "bring them up in the discipline and instruction of the Lord" (Ephesians 6:4). Think about your own interpretation of this and how you can fulfill this calling.

Your newborn's early years present a special chance for spiritual bonding. Strong methods to start this bond are to pray over your child, dedicate them to God, and share your wishes and blessings for their life. This spiritual bond demonstrates your dedication to being a godly role model for your child and lays the groundwork for their spiritual path.

It is customary to give thanks and pray throughout the first few days and weeks after the birth. Thank God for your child's safe arrival as well as your partner's health and strength. Ask for guidance in addressing the additional duties that come with being a parent. When making decisions that will impact your child's future, seek God's wisdom.

Your everyday routine is significantly altered by the birth of a child. Recognize that these adjustments are a necessary component of God's plan for your family and accept them with compassion and patience. This new season includes the learning curve of caring for a newborn, the new routines, and the restless nights. To find joy in the midst of these changes and to adapt to them, rely on God's knowledge and strength.

The arrival of a child may also have an effect on your marriage. Maintaining your relationship with your spouse and showing them love and support while you both get used to your new duties as parents is crucial. Talk honestly about your emotions, difficulties, and pleasures. Recall that your relationship is the cornerstone of your family and that it is essential to your child's wellbeing that you take care of this connection.

Your child's birth is a spiritual milestone in addition to a biological one. It is the start of a journey filled with love, support, and nurturing that lasts a lifetime. Open your heart to this new chapter and prepare to enjoy all that motherhood has to offer—challenges as well as blessings.

The Role of a Christian Father

This job includes more than just caring for and shielding your child; it also includes nurturing, teaching, and leading them in a way that is consistent with the beliefs and ideals of your religion.

Let's examine the different facets of this position and how you might live them out on your fathering journey.

Setting an example of love and compassion akin to Christ is a fundamental responsibility of a Christian father. You should emulate Jesus' grace, kindness, and patience in all that you say, do, and be. Your child is being modeled from the moment of their birth. Galatians 5:22–23 lists the fruits of the Spirit as love, joy, peace, patience, kindness, goodness, faithfulness, gentleness, and self-control. These are qualities that can be shown in every contact. Adopt these virtues and demonstrate to your child what it means to lead a life based on Christian love by doing so.

Teaching your child the morals and values described in the Bible is another crucial part of your job. Instead of beginning with structured teachings or memorizing passages from the Bible, this teaching begins with casual exchanges and discussions. Share biblical wisdom in real-world situations by telling tales, responding to inquiries about God and the religion, or setting an example of how to treat people with respect and kindness.

Lead your family in prayer and worship as a Christian parent. Establish rituals such as sharing in worship together, reading Bible stories, and having family prayer time. These rituals foster your child's spiritual development while fortifying the spiritual ties that bind your family together. Recall what Jesus said in Matthew 18:20, "I am with them wherever two or three gather in my name."

Establishing a household where God's presence is sensed and cherished depends on your leadership in these areas.

Providing discernment and spiritual advice is a major duty. Your child will grow up, be exposed to different influences, and be able to make decisions for themselves. Be there to mentor them, providing insight and biblical wisdom. The wisdom to "start children off on the way they should go, and even when they are old they will not turn from it" is emphasized in Proverbs 22:6. Your direction will assist them in making biblically-based decisions and navigating life's obstacles.

Establish an atmosphere of grace and forgiveness in your house. Instill in your child the value of forgiveness as a cornerstone of the Christian faith—both receiving and offering it. In your interactions, act with grace, demonstrating to your child that mistakes are not only to be punished or reprimanded but also opportunities for learning and development.

When parenting, collaborate carefully with your spouse to make sure your approaches to raising your child in faith are in line. Encourage one another, talk about effective parenting techniques, and decide together on the best ways to raise your child with Christian principles. Establishing a consistent and supportive atmosphere for your child is reliant on your participation in parenting.

Realize that God has given you one of the most important and transformative roles of your life. It's a path that calls for love, tolerance, direction, and a strong dedication to sharing and practicing your beliefs. As you take on this position, know that God will provide you with all you need to fulfill your calling as a parent.

Bonding With Your Newborn

This relationship is very important because it establishes your child's foundation for faith and molds their early perceptions of God's love and presence. Creating this connection requires deliberate behaviors and acts that both demonstrate your faith and ask God to be a part of your child's life.

There are a lot of opportunities for spiritual connection during the early days with your newborn. Even seemingly insignificant things can have a big impact, including praying over your child, leading praise songs or hymns, or even reading Scripture aloud to them as they sleep in your arms. These rituals not only calm and soothe your infant, but they also start the process of introducing God into their lives and their language.

The foundation of spiritual unity is prayer. Pray often for your child's well-being, development, and future. Add blessing prayers, pleading with God to lead them all the days of their lives. Say a little prayer of gratitude and protection over your infant while you hold them. These prayer times are more than just spiritual customs; they are an expression of your sincere wishes and dreams for your child's life, given to God in His tender care.

Baptism or dedication rituals are common Christian customs that serve as a ceremonial introduction of a child to the church. These rituals signify a promise to God and the church to raise your kid in accordance with Christian principles; they are more than merely symbolic actions. Think about organizing a dedication or baptism so that your church can join you in honoring and celebrating the spiritual journey your child is taking.

You have the chance to set an example of faith in your child's everyday interactions. They will learn more from your actions than from your words as they get older. Let your deeds - your generosity, tolerance, affection, and faith in God - serve as the first examples of faith kids encounter. Recall that you are your child's first and most important role model for living a religious life.

As your child gets older, include religion in your everyday activities. Simple acts like saying grace before meals, praying before bed, or reading aloud from the Bible can do this. By creating a smooth and natural foundation for your child's spiritual development, these rituals aid in normalizing the presence of faith in day-to-day living.

The spiritual tie that your child has with your partner is equally significant. Encourage and assist your spouse in discovering their own means of establishing a spiritual bond with your child. Ensure that you both actively participate in fostering your child's faith by sharing the role of spiritual leader in the family.

Lastly, keep in mind that developing a spiritual bond with your child is a group effort as much as an individual one. Engage your child's church community, friends, and extended family in their spiritual development. Your child's experience of faith can be enhanced by the guidance, knowledge, and feeling of community that this group can offer.

This is only the beginning of a journey that will grow and change over time. As you guide your child down their journey of faith, embrace each step with love, tolerance, and prayer, and put your trust in God's direction. One of the most meaningful and rewarding parts of being a parent is this journey, which is full of exciting, challenging, and growth-oriented experiences for both you and your child.

Guiding Light - Devotional

The birth of your child is a miraculous event, a tangible manifestation of life's wonder and God's grace. It brings to life the words of Psalm 127:3, where children are described as a heritage from the Lord, a reward from Him. As you hold your newborn, feeling the weight of this immense blessing, you embark on a path of nurturing, guiding, and loving this tiny soul.

In these moments, the essence of Ephesians 6:4 becomes your guide, reminding you of your duty to bring up your child in the Lord's discipline and instruction. This isn't just about the physical care but also about fostering a spiritual foundation, planting seeds of faith, hope, and love. Reflect on how you can live out this calling, embodying the values of the gospel in your everyday actions and interactions.

The initial years of your child's life offer a unique opportunity for spiritual bonding. This connection begins with small yet significant gestures—praying over your child, dedicating them to God, and sharing your hopes and blessings. These acts of faith lay the groundwork for their spiritual journey and reflect your commitment to being a godly example.

In the days and weeks that follow, turn your heart in gratitude and prayer. Thank God for the safe arrival of your child, and seek His guidance as you navigate the new responsibilities of parenthood.

Embrace the changes in your daily routine as part of God's plan, finding strength and joy in His wisdom.

Heavenly Father, lead us in raising our child with love, patience, and wisdom. Bless our family with Your grace and strengthen our faith through every step of this journey. Amen.

11

Growing Together

As you begin the eleventh month of your child's life—a period of early spiritual nurturing in addition to physical growth—it becomes increasingly clear that you have a duty to inculcate faith. Starting with these fragile early stages of development, we'll look at practical strategies to raise your child in the Christian faith in this chapter.

A life of faith is built on prayer, and starting your child off with this habit at a young age can have a significant positive impact. Begin with brief prayers before meals or before going to bed. Pray in a grateful and blessing-filled whisper to your infant as you rock or hold them. This not only establishes a prayer practice but also introduces your child to the idea of communicating with God at a young age. Recall that the meaning behind the words matters more than their eloquence.

Telling your child biblical stories is a great method to teach them to Christian values. Start with Bible storybooks for young children, emphasizing tales that highlight the goodness of God, the splendor of creation, and fundamental biblical principles. To keep the narrative interesting as you read, utilize emotive tones. This approach aims to establish connections through common religious narratives rather than only imparting knowledge about religion.

The atmosphere in your house is very important in helping your child grow in their faith. Make a place where faith is palpable and evident. One way to do this would be to incorporate Christian-themed décor, such as prayer corners or wall quotations. Play worship music or hymns that evoke awe and tranquility in your house. The intention is for faith to become a normal and constant part of your child's surroundings.

Youngsters pick up a lot of knowledge from observation. One of the most potent testimonies is to live out your faith in all that you do. Allow your youngster to witness you praying, reading the Bible, and modeling Christian characteristics like forgiveness, kindness, and patience. They learn from this example that faith is a vibrant, active aspect of day-to-day existence.

Seek to include your child's beliefs into daily practices as they get older. This can be accomplished by reciting brief Bible passages aloud as a group or through songs or prayers. Use these opportunities to teach your child about the significance and background of Christian festivals and celebrate them with fervor and passion.

In your home, prayer should be a constant topic of discussion. Even if your child is too small to comprehend or react, you should still pray with them. Allow them to hear your prayers for their future, for wisdom in parenting them, and for their general well-being. Encourage children to participate in prayer as they get older, offering their own praises and thanks to God.

Your child's spiritual development might be considerably enhanced by being a part of a church community. Participate in church activities, attend services on a regular basis, and interact with other Christian families. Through this activity, your child is exposed to a variety of Christian expressions and gains a sense of belonging to a broader church community.

This time is essential for laying the groundwork for a lifetime of spiritual growth. Seize every chance to strengthen their faith, aware that these preliminary actions serve as foundation for their eventual spiritual development and comprehension.

Adjusting to parenthood with God's Guidance

Being a parent can be an exciting and difficult journey, particularly in the beginning. It becomes imperative that you rely on God's direction as you move through this new role. This part will discuss how you can stay grounded spiritually and still adapt to the demands and changes of motherhood with the support of your faith, enabling you to provide your kid the best possible care.

Your life will undoubtedly change significantly when you become a parent—from new duties to changed sleep patterns. Accept these adjustments with confidence, knowing that God has prepared you for this position. Philippians 4:13, "I can do all this through Him who gives me strength," comes to mind. This verse can serve as a source of inspiration, serving as a reminder that you can overcome the difficulties of motherhood with God's assistance.

Being a parent might often involve making too many decisions. Seek guidance from God at these times. James 1:5 exhorts believers to approach God for wisdom since He freely offers it to everyone without pointing out flaws. Seek God's help while making decisions about your child's care, your techniques of punishment, or how to manage work and family obligations. When deciding what's best for your family, prayer can be a really useful tool.

Parenting may be stressful, especially in the beginning. An essential tool for handling this stress is prayer. In prayer, bring your worries and fears to God, and take solace in His presence.

"Cast all your anxiety on Him because He cares for you," says 1 Peter 5:7. Use prayer to gain comfort and assurance in God's love and care, rather than only to ask for assistance.

Being understanding and patient are essential qualities in fatherhood. Your tolerance will be put to the test at times—from restless nights to the difficulties of a developing child. Trust God to help you develop these qualities. The qualities of God's chosen people, such as kindness and patience, are described in Colossians 3:12. Make an effort to act like this while you are with your partner and child.

When parenting with a spouse, it's critical that you cooperate and support one another. Mutual understanding, communication, and shared duties are essential. Find methods to improve your bond when you embark on this new journey and support one another in your different duties as parents. Your partnership can be guided by Ephesians 4:2–3, which talks about bearing with one another in love while remaining modest, gentle, and patient.

Finding a balance between your personal needs, taking care of your child, and other obligations is another aspect of adjusting to motherhood. Taking care of oneself and keeping up a strong spiritual life are crucial. Maintain your own spiritual diet by participating in Bible study, fellowship, and private prayer. Recalling Christ's invitation to find rest in Him is crucial for new parents who may be feeling overwhelmed (Matthew 11:28–30).

During this time, your faith community can be a very helpful resource. Never be afraid to ask other believers for counsel, support, or hands-on assistance. The community can provide one a more comprehensive viewpoint as well as a feeling of support and belonging. "Carry each other's burdens, and in this way you will fulfill the law of Christ," as it states in Galatians 6:2. Include the people in your church family in your network of support.

Recognize that God is with you at every turn as you embrace this new chapter. You will experience the happiness and satisfaction that come with becoming a parent if you rely on Him for support, direction, and serenity.

Reflections on Fatherhood and Faith

Now let's consider how fatherhood and faith interact. The spiritual and parenting paths converge at this significant crossroads, each growing and enhancing the other. A deeper and more satisfying experience in both areas can result from knowing how parenthood and religion interact.

Being a father is a spiritual journey rather than just a biological or social position. It entails providing for a child's spiritual as well as their physical and emotional requirements. As you work to teach biblical truths and serve as an example of Christ-like love, this journey can strengthen your own faith. Fatherhood's difficulties and rewards frequently result in a greater comprehension of God's nature, including His unwavering love, tolerance, forgiveness, and direction. Consider how becoming a father has affected or illuminated your relationship with God.

Your religious beliefs act as a road map for your parenting endeavors. It offers a framework for comprehending the world, consolation during trying times, and guidelines for parenting. Your faith can provide you with comfort and perspective as you go through the highs and lows of fatherhood. Verses such as Proverbs 22:6, which advises raising children in the correct way, become more than just verses in the Bible—they become experiences.

Being a father can have a significant effect on your faith. It frequently results in a stronger sense of accountability, a keener understanding of the necessity of seeking God's direction, and a revitalized dedication to leading a life that exemplifies Christian principles. A child's utter dependency and fragility can serve as a powerful reminder of your own helplessness before God, encouraging humility and a stronger faith in His providence.

Experiencing the path of faith with your child is one of the most delightful aspects of being a Christian parent. This sharing is more than just imparting knowledge; it's being there for them as they come to know and develop their faith. Honor their spiritual accomplishments, be there for them when they have concerns about God, and help them navigate life's obstacles with sound biblical guidance. You have the profound privilege and trust of playing a part in their spiritual formation.

It is impossible to overestimate the importance of your church community in helping you on your fathering journey. Be in the company of other Christians who can provide knowledge, inspiration, and support. Participate in the family events, parenting programs, and men's groups that your church offers. These relationships can foster a sense of community and shared experience, as well as strength and direction.

Realize that your spiritual journey and your experience as a father are inextricably intertwined, with each enhancing and influencing the other. Remember that the things you have learned, grown stronger, and experienced on this trip will not only influence you going forward, but will also have a long-lasting effect on your child.

12

A Year of Blessings

It's a great accomplishment to reach the twelfth month of your fatherhood journey; it deserves contemplation and celebration. You probably experienced a mix of blessings and problems throughout your first year of parenthood, all of which shaped your experience and development as a parent. Together, we will examine the past year's journey, recognizing the happiness, the lessons discovered, and the ways that becoming a parent has improved your life.

A significant amount of personal growth frequently occurs during the first year of parenting. Think back on the happy and fulfilling times in your life. Maybe it was the first smile your baby gave you, or their first steps, or just the peaceful times you spent cuddling with them. The joys of fatherhood are brought to light by each of these significant anniversaries.

The obstacles you overcame are equally significant. Even though they can be challenging, going through the earliest stages of parenthood, having restless nights, and juggling work and family obligations can all result in tremendous personal development. They impart lessons in tolerance, forbearance, comprehension, and a greater capacity for love. Consider the ways in which these difficulties have molded you—not just as a father, but also as a person.

Give thanks for the experience of the past year for a moment. Experiencing the blessings of life as well as the difficulties of God might increase your gratitude. "Children are a heritage from the Lord, offspring a reward from him," according to Psalm 127:3. Consider becoming a father a blessing and a calling, and express gratitude for the chance to raise and mentor a child.

The first year of fatherhood is not just about your child's development but also about your own. Think about the ways that the last year has seen you progress. In what ways has your knowledge of God expanded? What changes in priorities have you made? In what ways has your ability to love and be patient grown? These introspection can provide light on the never-ending path of fatherhood and personal growth.

You probably needed your faith to help you get through the first year of parenthood. Consider how your faith has influenced your choices, given you solace during trying times, and made happy memories at happy occasions. Think about how your relationship with God has changed over time and how this relationship has affected the way you approach fatherhood.

Being a parent is a shared experience, and your partner's help during the first year is priceless. Think back on the ways that having a child has helped you both, brought you closer, and taught you lessons. Recognize your partner's accomplishments and selflessness, and think about ways you may build on these qualities in the years to come.

In the journey of parenthood, the support of a community is crucial, be it family, friends, or a faith community. Consider the assistance you've had and the ways in which it has influenced your experience. Your sense of community and belonging can be strengthened by acknowledging and being grateful for this support.

As you celebrate reaching this one-year mark, now is the perfect time to look ahead. What aspirations do you have for the future of your child? What changes do you see coming in your role as a father? What morals and teachings do you want your child to learn as they grow up? Your path forward and the course of your fatherhood adventure beyond this first year can be shaped by these reflections.

Continuing Your Spiritual Journey as a Father

Your child's faith and comprehension should develop together with them. This never-ending path is about more than just parenting; it's about strengthening your own spiritual foundation, developing your child's faith, and setting an example for them.

Growing up and starting to experience the world with your child gives you a chance to develop your beliefs as well. Spend some time learning new things about your faith from your child's perspective. Their amazement, curiosity, and innocence might provide new insights into well-known spiritual ideas or biblical stories. Accept these times as chances for research and progress in mutual spirituality.

Your child's innate curiosity about the world, especially spiritual things, will grow as they move into new developmental stages. Be ready to respond according to their age and comprehension to their inquiries concerning God, faith, and the Bible. Take use of these questions to explore your beliefs further, possibly going back to review parts of your own spiritual knowledge that may require clarification or affirmation.

It's crucial to keep up regular spiritual activities both for your own development and to establish a routine for your family. Keep up the worship, Bible reading, and family prayers. As your child gets older, include them in these activities more. You could, for example, encourage them to pray, engage in family Bible study, or lead praise music. These customs support the idea that faith is vital in day-to-day living.

Along with official instruction, your child will pick up Christian values from watching you live. Make an effort to embody Christian values such as forgiveness, kindness, patience, and love. Give examples of how to practice honesty, compassion, and service to others as methods to live out your beliefs. Your behavior will reveal a lot about the values you uphold and want your child to learn.

It's important to keep growing your own faith even though you'll be spending a lot of time developing your child's. Maintain your dedication to your individual spiritual practices, such as Bible study, prayer, and communion with other believers. These practices will prepare you to be the spiritual leader your family needs and are essential to your spiritual well-being.

There is no doubt that becoming a parent will bring problems that need for discernment and wisdom. Seek God's direction in order to overcome these obstacles. Scriptures that encourage believers to ask God for wisdom, such as James 1:5, serve as a constant reminder that we can always turn to God for direction. This knowledge will support you not only in decision-making as a parent but also in knowing how to navigate challenging circumstances in a way that honors your beliefs.

Establish and preserve a religious culture in your household. The morals you follow, the discussions you have, the media you select, and the way you engage with one another all contribute to creating this culture. Create a space in your house where faith is not just taught but actually experienced and lived.

Maintaining your involvement in a religious community is crucial for both you and your offspring. Participating in fellowship groups, service initiatives, and church events gives one a sense of accountability and community. Additionally, it gives your child a more comprehensive understanding of Christianity by exposing them to a variety of ways that faith is demonstrated.

Your faith journey will change as your child grows. Recognize that your spiritual needs and understanding may vary throughout time, and be open to this progression. Accept fresh approaches to growing closer to God and strengthening your faith. Your child will benefit from this openness as well as the flexible and rich spiritual environment it offers.

Gratitude and Hope For the Future

Being a father is an ongoing journey with new delights and challenges every day. It's important to take a moment to reflect on the journey thus far and to look forward with hope and faith. The significance of thankfulness, looking forward to future achievements, and the ongoing path of spiritual development and fatherhood will all be covered in this part.

When you look back on the previous year, count all of the blessings—big and small—that have accompanied your journey to becoming a father. Celebrate the victories, the times you spend connecting with your child, and the strengthening ties that unite your family. Thank God for his wisdom, your partner's support, the affection of your extended family, and your religion community. Gratitude is fostered by acknowledging these blessings, as Psalm 136:1 tells us to "Give thanks to the Lord, for He is good." His love is eternal.

There are a lot of things you should be prepared for and hope for in your child's future. Every growth stage will present fresh encounters and chances to mentor, care for, and instruct. Every developmental milestone, like as their first words, steps, or preschool entry, offers an opportunity to see how their distinct personality and abilities emerge. Aim to be present and involved in these upcoming times with enthusiasm.

Your function as a spiritual guide becomes more crucial as your child gets older. It is your honor to lead them throughout these early years, providing a solid spiritual basis that will influence how they view the world. Along with giving kids biblical lessons and tales, this mentoring program also teaches children how to apply their faith in real-world situations. Keep praying for discernment and direction in this capacity, having faith that God will provide you with the necessary tools.

This is not the conclusion of your spiritual and personal development journey. Maintain your quest for personal development, realizing that your spiritual well-being has a direct bearing on your capacity to guide and provide for your family. Take part in activities that strengthen your relationship with God, such fellowship, study, and prayer. Accept chances for education and development, realizing that fatherhood is a dynamic position that changes as your child does.

One cannot stress the importance of a nurturing community in a child's upbringing. Keep participating in church activities and seek out advice, inspiration, and support from other Christians. Give your kids the opportunity to discover the benefits of belonging to a faith-based community, where they can form deep connections and learn from a variety of role models.

Being a father is a journey that has its share of pleasures and hardships. Accept that there will be challenging times ahead, as well as periods of great happiness and satisfaction. See every obstacle as a chance to improve and advance as a parent and a disciple of Christ.

Encourage your youngster to have faith and optimism as you lead them. Instill in them the optimism that comes from knowing that God is always at work, even in the most trying situations.

Encourage their faith by teaching them about God's love and grace and how it affects their lives.

AFTERWORD

As we approach the end of this book, it is critical to understand that the journey of Christian fatherhood is not over and is not limited to the first year of your child's life. Rather, it's a lifetime dedication, a long journey that combines your child's growth with your own spiritual and personal development. Every day on this journey offers a fresh chance to live out your faith, cultivate love, and mentor your child using Christian values.

Being a father is a constantly changing role, with new delights and challenges at every turn in your child's development. Your ability to understand, be patient, and show love will all increase as they do. From toddlerhood to adolescence and beyond, embrace every stage as a chance to strengthen your bond with your child and your connection with God. Never forget that there is always something to learn and an opportunity to deepen your faith in every circumstance, no matter how happy or difficult.

You continue to influence your child's spiritual development. As they get older, the seeds of faith that were sown in their early years will require watering, nurturing, and perhaps pruning. Their perception of God and their connection with Him will be significantly impacted by your dedication to practicing your faith, imparting biblical knowledge, and setting a high example. Remember that each person's spiritual path is distinct and special, so exercise patience and perseverance.

The nature of your relationship will change as your child grows. Be ready to gracefully adjust to these changes. Your child will require your assistance at times as a teacher, friend, mentor, or just a sympathetic ear. Pray to God for the discernment to see these needs and the adaptability to provide for them. Your capacity for adaptation will improve your faith and character in addition to strengthening your bond with your child.

Your faith has an impact on those outside of your own family. It affects your church, your neighborhood, and eventually, society at large. You are leaving a legacy that will last when you are gone by raising a child in the faith. This snowball effect is a potent illustration of how crucial your job as a Christian father is.

The most crucial thing to keep in mind is that you are not traveling alone. God is always with you, providing consolation, support, and strength. Rely on Him during uncertain times, celebrate with Him during happy ones, and seek His guidance for all of your decisions. Being a father is, at its core, a journey you share with God.

Look forward and greet the future with trust and hope. Being a Christian father is a wonderful, difficult, and fulfilling journey. It's a journey that molds not just your child's life but also your own. Proceed with the lessons learned in this first year, understanding that every day is a gift and a chance to practice your faith, show your child love, and lead him in the ways of the Lord.

Finally, find comfort in the fact that becoming a Christian parent has been one of the most significant and life-changing experiences of your life. It has the capacity to bring about great happiness, meaningful connection, and spiritual fulfillment. May you believe in God's direction and supply at every turn, walking this path with self-assurance, love, and a growing faith.